Ana Claudia Moutella Pimenta

Pathographs of Dental Mutilates

Ana Claudia Moutella Pimenta

Pathographs of Dental Mutilates

Dental Mutilation Pathographies

ScienciaScripts

Imprint

Any brand names and product names mentioned in this book are subject to trademark, brand or patent protection and are trademarks or registered trademarks of their respective holders. The use of brand names, product names, common names, trade names, product descriptions etc. even without a particular marking in this work is in no way to be construed to mean that such names may be regarded as unrestricted in respect of trademark and brand protection legislation and could thus be used by anyone.

Cover image: www.ingimage.com

This book is a translation from the original published under ISBN 978-613-9-62081-4.

Publisher:
Sciencia Scripts
is a trademark of
Dodo Books Indian Ocean Ltd. and OmniScriptum S.R.L publishing group

120 High Road, East Finchley, London, N2 9ED, United Kingdom
Str. Armeneasca 28/1, office 1, Chisinau MD-2012, Republic of Moldova, Europe
Printed at: see last page
ISBN: 978-620-7-71228-1

SUMMARY

DEDICATORY

To those who haven't had opportunities in life to make their dreams come true.

ACKNOWLEDGMENTS

Where do we start to say thank you?

To God, who through grace, caring for each one of us, has placed me where I am, with joys and sorrows, dilemmas and hopes, in order to understand my role in life's journey.

Every single member of my family, who made sure that my achievements and accomplishments were possible.

To my son, who provided all the technical and emotional support to make this work possible.

To my friend Luciane Pezzato, who gave me all the support and encouragement I needed for this doctorate.

To my advisor Solange L'Abbate, who generously agreed to guide me.

To each of the patients who shared their stories.

To everyone who believed.

To everyone who cheered.

SUMMARY

The aim of this research was to analyze the process of institutionalization of a dental prosthesis service in the municipality of Campinas/SP, taking into account the municipality's health policy, the structuring of services and care practices in the face of oral health needs from the point of view of the patient-subject. The theoretical and methodological approach is based on Institutional Analysis, and the research tools used were diaries kept by the researcher and interviews with mutilated SUS dental users in the eastern region of the municipality in question, with the aim of developing their *pathographic histories.* The concept of *pathography* relates to the ways in which individuals affected by serious illnesses try to order events, producing narratives in which causal attributions, motivations and the roles of the agents causing the illnesses are established. Institutional Analysis seeks to understand a given social and organizational reality based on the discourses and practices of the subjects. It is therefore hoped that, through pathographies, institutional analysis and the concept of bucality (social work carried out by the mouth), we can identify the objective and subjective dimensions of patients with dental mutilation who have used, are using or are still waiting to use the service, understanding the work process within the current context, analyzing the potential and difficulties from the point of view of the patient-subjects, pointing out possibilities for qualification in the micro-work spaces.

Keywords: Oral Health; Institutional Analysis,

Pathographies and Orality.

PRESENTATION:

We are going to travel a long way along the road of *Collective Health*, the north of which is the *Unified Health System*, passing through *Family Health*, actually the *Family Health Strategy*, in an attempt to achieve *Oral Health* as a relevant part of general health, in the direction of integrality. We chose to go through *Primary Care*, as recommended by the Ministry of Health in the *National Oral Health Policy*, although sometimes we may be in *Secondary Care*. The aim here is to try to understand the meaning that people give to the different aspects of their existential reality, based on the assumption that each person processes different meanings about the dimensions of their lives, according to their personal experiences and the specific contexts in which they are inserted. In this way, we hope to reach the individuals who are the subjects of their own stories and who will tell us their *pathological stories.* To do this, we ask for permission from *bucality* and *subjectivity to* try to produce care in the daily life of the services, observing the events, situations, manifestations and details that are part of day-to-day life. *Institutional Analysis* will be our food for thought along the way and, of course, we're going to be attentive, keep an eye on the ball, make sure we don't miss any *Analyzers,* without forgetting to drink water to hydrate our *implication,* which mustn't dry up and turn into *over-implication...* Let's start by recalling a little of the history of *Collective Health*, its antecedents, the process of creating ABRASCO and the *institutionalization of the SUS*. The creation of *the Family Health Teams* as a national health policy strategy and the inclusion of oral health teams. From then on, *"Smiling Brazil"* opened up space for the rehabilitation of patients with *mutilated teeth* and it is here that I begin to interact with history, when I become responsible for a prosthesis service that dialogues with the lives of *edentulous users* and, for that, it is impossible not to be *involved.* We're all involved! I'm going to listen to the speeches, understand the feelings and share a little of the stories told by these subjects in the interviews, in order to put together their *pathographies*. Finally, I'll discuss the findings and try to produce a synthesis, an analysis that will lead us towards thoughts, reflections, *encounters* and, who knows, *instituting* movements.

INTRODUCTION

1.1 Historical Background of Health: from "Religious Explanations" to Collective Health in Brazil

For a long time, man has been concerned with finding explanations for illness and healing. In each period of human history, different meanings have been given to the health-disease process.

In the religious era in which writing had not been created, man generally lived in nomadic tribes. Illness was related to a higher power, a disharmony with the cosmic order, and treatments consisted of witchcraft rituals and exorcism. Archaeologists have unearthed human skulls that had been pierced by healers so that the evils would leave the patient's body. Teas, herbs, infusions and other empirical methods were used to treat illnesses (Oliveira and Egry, 2000[1] ; Giudice, 2008[2] ; Fadel and Saliba, 2010).[3]

With the development of cities, commerce, writing, the arts, architecture, painting and great thinkers emerged. Disease then came to be seen as the result of an imbalance between the four elements called humors - earth, water, air and fire (Oliveira and Egry, 2000[1]; Fadel and Saliba, 2010[3]).

Specifically in Brazil and in relation to oral health, Indians and blacks in the colonial period used their knowledge to deal with dental pain and suffering. The practices were based on rites that included prayers, herbs and procedures with rudimentary instruments (Narvai and Frazâo, 2008).[4]

Foucault (1984 p.82)[5] stated that "since the end of the 16th century and the beginning of the 17th century, all the nations of the European world have been concerned with the state of health of their population in a political, economic and scientific climate characteristic of the period dominated by mercantilism".

Fadel and Saliba (2010)[3] , say that if we go a little further back in history, we find Modern Medicine, which was on the one hand religious in nature, where there was a need for divine interference in the processes of healing and getting sick, and on the other, scientific thinking, based on knowledge of human anatomy.

For Foucault (1984)[5] , modern medicine was a social, individualistic medicine that valued the doctor-patient relationship. With the development of capitalism in the late 18th and early 19th centuries, the body was socialized as a force for production and work.

With the incessant search for explanations for the health-disease process came the development of biology, microbiology and, consequently, the discovery of disease-causing microorganisms in the mid-19th century, "when the belief in the model of scientific rationality as the only way to obtain the truth was consolidated". (Fadel and Saliba, 2010, p.522)[3] .

From the time of the Industrial Revolution in England and the development of urban structures in France, Social Medicine emerged, linking working conditions, housing, food, access to goods and services, including health, leisure and political participation, to strategies for transforming reality into health (Foucault, 1984[5] ; Fadel and Saliba, 2010)[3].

From Primitive Medicine or the Religious Era, through the Hippocratic Era, Modern Medicine, the Bacteriological Era, to Medicine

Socially, there have been transformations that have had an impact on populations. The "knowledge" produced by medicine over time has brought progressive knowledge of the body and illnesses and has managed to develop interventions capable of controlling damage, relieving suffering and pain and prolonging life, but this limited form of health practice has been questioned for some years now. For some, the biomedical model has failed. Care has acquired other meanings because the health-disease process is not reduced to the biological (Campos, 2003[6] ; Giudice, 2008).[2]

A new paradigm in the 1970s and 1980s highlighted the association between living conditions and health, which is no longer understood as the mere absence of disease, but as the result of a set of individual and collective, historical, social, economic, ethnic, religious, cultural, psychological, labor, biological and environmental factors, among others. (Fadel and Saliba, 2010)[3] . This research will address this type of explanation for the issues surrounding oral health.

Oliveira and Egry (2000)[1] , agree that other dimensions have been related to diseases that have come to be understood as multi-causal and, therefore, the need has arisen to value the genesis of multiple interrelated factors in causal networks, including individual well-being, individual perception of health and rescuing subjectivity, whether of the subject themselves or of the community.

In this context, Collective Health emerged in Brazil in the 1970s, as part of the Health Reform movement, which sought to articulate the different fields of health care. Gradually, the term "Collective Health" began to be used to refer to meetings, events, courses, departments, centers and research institutes, culminating in the founding of the Brazilian Association of Postgraduate Studies in Collective Health (ABRASCO) in 1979 (L'Abbate, 2013).[7]

Cecilia Donnangelo (1983)[8] defined Collective Health as "a set of tendencies to broaden and recompose the space for intervention or the field of knowledge and practice and noted that this gave rise to a different kind of academic production, mainly due to the use of instruments from the Social Sciences". (Donnangelo, 1983, p.19)[8]

L'Abbate, in the Introduction to the book "Anâlise Institucional & Saùde Coletiva" (2013)[7], states that this article by Donnangelo and the creation of ABRASCO constitute **the Founding Institutionalization of Collective Health** (original emphasis by the author), which brought an innovative/institutional character to the way of considering health in Brazil.

1.2 The SUS was created in 1988, the Family Health Program in 1994 and Oral Health was only included in 2000...

According to Fonsêca and Junqueira (2014)[9], the Health Reform was an intense political movement that mobilized Brazilian society to build health awareness and, as a result of the struggles undertaken, the right to health was guaranteed in the New Constitution of 1988. The demands began in the first half of the 1970s, when a growing process of privatization of health actions and services was underway. From then on, with the delineation of the Unified Health System, SUS, it was possible to articulate different social segments around a set of propositions synthesized in the slogan "for the democratization of health and society" and which achieved the unification of the system, the decentralization of actions (so that municipalities could make decisions at a local level), universal access and popular control.

Thus, we are living through a period of concretization of the 1988 Magna Carta, in which a new constitutional "status" has been granted to the municipalities (the only country in the world to do this) which, together with the states, have become autonomous constituent units of the federation.

The Eighth National Health Conference (CNS), held in Brasilia/DF in March 1986, was a privileged moment for political discussions and agreements, and its main resolutions were favorably received by the members of the National Constituent Assembly, so that when the Constitution of the Federative Republic of Brazil was promulgated, it established in its Title VIII of the Social Order: (a) Health as a right of all and a duty of the State (art. 196); (b) the creation of a Unified Health System - **SUS** (art. 198) (my emphasis); (c) decentralized management with command in each sphere of government (art. 198); (d) comprehensive actions with priority given to preventive measures (art. 198) and (e) community participation in decisions relating to health (art. 198). Later, in 1990, federal laws 8080 and 8142 came to regulate these constitutional precepts.

The Family Health Program (PSF), conceived and implemented in 1994, is the strategy used by the Ministry of Health to reorient the care model of the Unified Health System (SUS), starting with primary care. For the Ministry of Health, the Family Health Team (ESF) is the main tool for strengthening Brazilian primary care. This strategy began in June 1991 with the incorporation of Community Health Agents (ACS) and in 1994 the first family health teams were formed.

Calado (2002)[10] states that the PSF was a response by the Ministry of Health to the crisis experienced by the health sector in the last two decades.

According to the Ministry of Health, a family health unit is intended to "provide continuous care in basic specialties, with a multi-professional team qualified to carry out health promotion, protection and recovery activities, characteristic of the primary level of care" (Brazil, 2006)[11] .

It is known that primary care units should be able to solve most of the health problems of their communities, providing quality care, avoiding unnecessary hospitalizations and improving the quality of life of the population. Thus, this level of care represents the main "gateway", the first contact with the health services and should be organized through referrals and counter-referrals to the other levels of the system (Brasil, 2004[12] ; Brasil, 2006)[11] but, in this research, we will discuss some of the difficulties facing these guidelines, which are still far from being achieved, due to the crisis that the SUS is going through in the current context.

The legislation states that the Family Health Program must choose the family as the target social nucleus in a defined territory and add the principles of social responsibility, interdisciplinarity and intersectorality, as well as health surveillance. Primary Care, on the other hand, must be a service of high quality and resolubility, it must value health promotion and protection and, finally, it must be part of a hierarchical system so that the objectives of the Family Health Program can be met. (Brasil, 2004)[12]

Oral Health was only included in this model after the publication of Ordinance 1.444 of 28/12/2000. Since then, 12 years after the "creation" of the SUS, there has been a huge gap in the inclusion of oral health in the system. Only since 2000 (Ordinance 267 of 06/03/2001) has there been approval and financial incentive for Oral Health, linked to the creation of Oral Health Teams (ESB) within the Family Health Program (PSF), created in 1994 (Brasil, 2000).[13]

Frazâo and Narvai (2009, p.64)[14] state that "since the creation of the SUS in 1988, the inclusion of oral health has been marked by conflicts and contradictions, expressing the different projects in dispute in Brazilian society". Until then, there were only centralized and vertical dental programs aimed at schoolchildren and workers registered with the social security system.

Fonsêca and Junqueira (2014)[9] agree and state that for a long time the oral health system established in the public service was characterized by procedures provided in an unsystematic manner, with free demand and marked by mutilating techniques, based on the complaint-conduct.

The document that defined the foundations of the Family Health Program states that, in opposition to the traditional model, centered on the disease and the hospital, priority would be given to actions to promote and protect the health of individuals, whether adults, children or the elderly, healthy or sick, in an integral way, as stated by Baldani, Fadel, Possamai and Queiroz in 2005[16] .

In 2006, the PSF ceased to be a program and was accredited as a Family Health Strategy (ESF) through Ordinance No. 648 of March 28, 2006. The idea was to turn the PSF into a permanent and ongoing strategy, since the program has a fixed timeframe.

Thus, the ESF is a strategy for reorienting the health care model from primary care, with a proposal to change the model centered on the doctor and the hospital to a model focused on comprehensive care, where the user is inserted within their socioeconomic and cultural community, establishing the recognition of health as a right of citizenship, evidenced by the improvement of living conditions through more resolute, comprehensive and humanized services.

Ferraz and Leite (2016)[17] define the PSF as the Family Health Strategy (ESF), because the terminology of the program points to an activity with a beginning, development and end. The ESF reorganizes primary care and relies on programmatic activities and periodic evaluations.

Still according to these authors, the ESF pointed to a change in the focus of care, which began to have the family as its center, assisted (when necessary) in its social space (assigned area), with its singularities, by a multi-professional team, aiming at more resolutive and integrative practices, with epidemiology as the structuring axis of actions.

The fact that dentistry is not included in this first stage appears to be a contradiction in terms, according to Ferraz and Leite (2016)[17] , since prevention, promotion, treatment and rehabilitation actions in health should include oral health, since the latter is part of health as a whole and should not be fragmented from other services.

It is worth noting that since the First National Oral Health Conference (CNSB) in 1986, there has been a proposal to include oral health in the SUS, through a "National Oral Health Program", although it was not accepted by the governments that followed (Narvai and Frazao, 2008)4.

The Second National Oral Health Conference, held in 1993, approved guidelines and political strategies in the country, recognizing oral health as a *right to citizenship (emphasis added)* and indicated a new model of care and human resources necessary to guarantee universal access and equity in dental care (Narvai and Frazao, 2008).[4]

After seven years between the first and second CNSB - 1986 and 1993, another seven years passed and a new perspective for the National Oral Health Policy was opened in 2000, with the issuance of Ordinance 1444 of 28/12/2000, by the Ministry of Health, establishing a financial incentive for the reorganization of oral health care. (Calado, 2002)[10]

Today, the National Primary Care Policy (PNAB) defines oral health as one of the strategic areas for the operationalization of Primary Care throughout the country. In addition, the PNAB establishes competencies between the federated entities, financing modalities, attributions of the strategy's professionals, including oral health professionals, and thus creates conditions for the consolidation of oral health in the ESF.

The Ministry of Health outlines guidelines for the ESB to follow the principles and regulations of the SUS in order to seek greater access for the population to oral health actions, integrating the service network and establishing a referral and counter-referral system that increases resolutiveness and allows users to be monitored. The replacement of traditional practices will be achieved to the extent that they follow the characteristics advocated by the ESF, which are: client targeting, comprehensive care, connection with medium and high complexity care, prioritization of the family as the central axis of care, humanization, multidisciplinary care, development of preventive and health promotion actions, participation and social control, permanent and continuing education, planning actions, evaluation and permanent monitoring of the teams. In addition to all this, planning should be done in the logic of strategic planning, allowing for the prioritization of cases and the organization of clinical care. (Brasil, 2000)

Viana, Martelli and Pimentel (2011)[18] believe that throughout this period there has been an exponential growth in the implantation of ESBs in the ESF, but little has been done to monitor this increase. In addition, attention should be paid to the Brazilian reality, which faces the presence of strong social exclusion, bearing in mind that the economic measures and social policies implemented have not yet reduced the inequalities of a large portion of the Brazilian population, such as, in our case, the issue of edentulism[1] and its influence on people's oral health[2] and subjectivity.

---

1 Edentulism: absence of tooth(s)
2 Bucality: terminology created by Botazzo, 2000, which will be discussed in Chapter II.

CHAPTER I: THE AUTHOR'S PROFESSIONAL CAREER AND ITS IMPLICATIONS

Implication refers to the affective, existential and professional relationships that a person has with the institutions in which they work. These relationships involve different levels of closeness, friendship, partnership and ideology, generating different types of commitment. Implication is our involvement, sometimes even unconscious, with everything we do.

René Lourau states that the word "implication" has tended for some years to be used synonymously with other words such as commitment, participation, investment and motivation (2004 p.246)[19] . He also states that "they constitute value judgments about ourselves and others, intended to measure the degree of activism in a task or institution and the amount of time/money we devote to it, as well as the emotional charge invested" (2004 p.187) .[19]

Lourau defines implication as the relationship that the researcher has with the object of research and/or intervention.

Man's relationship with his life and the society in which he lives, "the subject at the heart of the social and political game", in whatever position he occupies, must try to understand the processes that surround him.

Guillier and Samson (1997, p. 19)[20] state that implications refer to links existing in the past that are updated in the present, in view of new contexts, and "constitute provisional agencies forming the transversality of a social form".

Lourau, *apud* L'Abbate 2013[7] , p. 47, reaffirms that implication is:

(...) the set of relationships that the intellectual refuses, consciously or not, to analyze in his practice, whether these are relationships with his objects of study, with the cultural institution, with his family environment, as well as with other dimensions, such as money, power, libido, and in general with the society of which he is a part.

Monceau (2008, p.22)[21] states that the implication exists even if we don't want it to. The question is not the quantity of the implication, but the intensity with which it operates in the subjects.

It is therefore a question of analyzing the mode of implication rather than its existence, or quantity of implication, since it cannot be measured in weight. (...) It is a question of understanding our mode of relationship with the institution because this implication has an effect even if we don't know it.

The concept of implication was introduced into Institutional Analysis[3] as one of the indispensable elements of a methodological theoretical project, both for research and intervention (Lourau, 2014)[22]. The ideology that today can be called "implicationist" had existed for some time, but the word "implication" had nothing to do with the old concept. The word "implication" was used to incorporate Freudian concepts of transference and countertransference into collective situations.

The notion of implication, for Lourau, is the "scandal of Institutional Analysis[3] ", as it calls into question the place of the so-called "experts", due to its destabilizing and denaturalizing character of comfortable and uncritically occupied places.

Georges Lapassade and René Lourau (1972)[23] in *Keys to Sociology,* defined the preliminary features of the notion of implication. However, it wasn't until 1973 that this concept became more explicit in their publications. With a view to building a new field of coherence, where research is not separated from intervention and where the field of intervention includes the researcher and the object of their research.

According to L'Abbate, 2013[7] , Lourau, throughout his work, questions the implications, since the implication denounces what the institution triggers in us: values, interests, expectations, desires, beliefs, among others that are imbricated in our personality.

Coimbra and Nascimento (2008, p. 145)[24] concluded that the analysis of implication brings feelings, perceptions, actions and events into the field of research. Therefore, they understand that "one is always implicated, since implication is not a matter of will, a conscious decision, a voluntary act. It is in

---

3 The concept of Institutional Analysis will be discussed in the Methodology.

the world, because it is a relationship that we always establish with the institutions we encounter, which constitute us and pass through us." In this way, the implicated researcher analyzes the place they occupy in society, in the social division of labour, in social relations in general and not just in the context of the intervention/research they are carrying out."

For Barbier (1985)[25] there are three dimensions to the concept of implication: psycho-affective, historical-existential and structural-professional. The same author (p.108) states that "the researcher is soon confronted with his psycho-affective implication because, in action research, the object of investigation always questions the foundations of the deep personality."

The psycho-affective dimension is the one that touches me the most, although this characteristic could lead me to over-implication, a term coined by Lourau (2004, p. 191)[19] , for whom:

Over-implication and activism, once analyzed, have extremely passive aspects: submission to explicit orders or implicit consignments of the new economic and social order, eager to fill the large gaps produced by both disaffection and institutionalization. (...) it also interferes with the analysis of implication when we isolate one of the fields of analysis, psychologizing it.

From an IA point of view, overimplication not only produces overwork, but also stress, illness and even death. According to Lourau (2004, p. 195)[19], "death by overwork shouldn't scare researchers who are overimplicated at work away from the concept of implication!"

But the affective dimension we were talking about is linked to the ideological and professional aspects, because I have always had an intense desire to (re)think my daily professional practice as a dentist, working for 26 years in the Unified Health System (SUS), 19 of them in the Municipal Health Department of Campinas/SP. Throughout this time, I have been looking for partnerships, interlocutions, relationships, paths... I've been trying to reflect on my involvement and over-involvement, problematizing the way I've been working, trying to understand how and where I want to go. It's essential that I can carry out this analysis in order to understand the forces that run through my work, so that I can understand how I've been working in the SUS and how I've been carrying out the dentistry in which I was trained.... I'm questioning whether my training coincides with my work or not, and why?

For Coimbra and Nascimento (2008, p.147)[24] it is essential that we undertake a constant, daily analysis of the places we occupy and the forces that cross us and affect us at different times. These authors consider the analysis of implication:

(...) it is a device, it is always micropolitical, it is always an analysis of our modes of existence which, according to Spinoza and Nietzsche, must be thought of from immanent criteria, without any appeal to transcendental values. Thus, the analysis of implications, being micropolitical, is found on the plane of immanence, on the plane of encounters where enunciations are produced, where "making seen and making spoken" are present. In other words, to use the analysis of implications is to make visible and audible the forces that cross us, affect us and constitute us on a daily basis.

Monceau (2010)[26] states that it is possible to try to transform an institution as long as we are inside it, analyzing its daily acts, devices and relationships. Still according to this author, the proposal for intervening in an institution is to work from what connects us to it, in other words, our involvement. The possible analysis is circumstantial and provisional, therefore, in this approach, "the researcher occupies a privileged place to analyze power relations, including those that permeate him", as stated by Romagnoli, (2014, p.46)[27] .

I'm currently a dental surgeon working in the Prosthesis Service at SUS/Campinas and I'm also a lecturer at the School of Dentistry at PUC-Campinas, where I graduated in 1990. I notice big differences compared to when I graduated. The training of dental professionals after the creation of the SUS began to involve other disciplines, to have another focus, other guidelines, other attributions, more coherent with the national reality. The curriculum is very different! The failure of the biomedical model, in force until then, required changes in public policies, with transformations in the training of professionals and in the health work process (Ferraz and Leite, 2016)[17].

According to the Report of the first National Conference on Oral Health, in 1986, the year I entered the Dentistry course, the professional practice model was only capable of covering 5% of the population, and was described as ineffective, inefficient, monopolizing, high-cost, high-tech, elitist, iatrogenic and mutilating.

The last few decades have seen changes not only in the curriculum at schools and universities, but also in the political, social and economic frameworks in our country. We've made a lot of progress, but the past of social and racial exclusion, as well as income distribution and difficulty in accessing essential goods and services, including health, are still insufficient for the entire population.

Ferraz and Leite (2016, p. 303)[17] state that "the great advance and, at the same time, the **challenge** (my emphasis) of Public Health in Brazil was its restructuring with the creation of the SUS in the Federal Constitution of 1988. In 1986, when I started dental school, we didn't yet have the current Constitution and today I find myself practicing my profession, most of the time, in this Health System that didn't exist at the time.

Professional dentists were prepared to work in a model that prioritized the treatment of dental diseases, in an autonomous way, without experience of teamwork, closely linked to technicality and tied to individual basic procedures. (Fonsêca and Junqueira, 2014)[9] .

However, despite the progress made by the SUS, the population is still marked by inequality and inequities and I feel I have an ethical commitment to question the different variables that involve my work and the situation experienced by the users I serve in the public service. So I set out from this challenge to question my involvement and, consequently, my work and how this is reflected in the service and the users I serve.

That's why, after graduating in Dentistry, I went on to specialize in Public Health at the Department of Preventive and Social Medicine, now the Department of Collective Health, at the Faculty of Medical Sciences (FCM), in 2001, and later on, in Public Health.

I did my Master's in the Department of Collective Health at the Piracicaba School of Dentistry (FOP) in 2007, both of which belong to Unicamp. I was trying to better understand the SUS, which was so recent and new to me.

After graduating in 1990, I took part in several public examinations, which were the only viable job options for me at the time.

of the municipality of Indaiatuba. I only cared for the children of a public school to which I had been assigned. Basically, I restored and extracted baby teeth and sometimes came across permanent teeth destroyed by caries. I stayed there until I applied for another job that would bring me closer to home, as I lived in Campinas. I joined the Social Service for Industry (SESI) and remained in this job until I passed another exam for a dentist, where I am today, in the Campinas City Hall.

I worked in various health centers, experienced different types of services, met professionals from different careers... After 10 years, I took part in an internal selection process and was selected to work at the Health Worker Education Center (CETS), believing that I would collaborate in the training of oral health technicians and/or assistants, but I soon realized that it was a very political position, in which we did the support or "Middle Function" between managers and employees, which caused me a lot of frustration. In 2006, when I received an invitation to become a reference for the Prosthesis Service in the Eastern District, I didn't hesitate to return to the service and, since then, I've been caring for edentulous patients[4] These users/subjects come to the prosthesis service for different reasons and in different ways, full of expectations and, during the process of making the prostheses (an estimated time of 5 sessions that can last up to 6 months), they show emotions and feelings that touched me. I began to try to understand the meaning that people give to the different aspects of their existential reality, based on the assumption that these individuals process different meanings about the dimensions of their lives and according to their personal experiences and the specific contexts in which they are inserted.

---

4 *Edentulous patients: patients without teeth*

These experiences gave rise to the desire to investigate this subject through a doctorate in Collective Health. This doctorate is related to another project I took part in called "Innovation in the Production of Oral Health Care: Possibilities for a New Approach in the Dental Clinic for the SUS"[5] , coordinated by Prof. Dr. Carlos Botazzo from USP's School of Public Health, whom I knew from books and articles and who interested me greatly, especially the concept of Bucality he developed. It was as if we spoke the same language, shared the same anxieties and wanted the same dentistry, which was very different from that for which we had been trained and which didn't contribute to solving the population's oral health problems.

This project included USP, São Paulo campus and Ribeirão Preto campus, as well as the University of Pernambuco, in Recife and the city of Campinas, where I was a researcher together with Prof[a] . Dr. Luciane Maria Pezzato who did the institutional supervision. It was an audacious, unique project that sought to innovate/renew traditional dentistry with new concepts and foundations. We'll come back to it later.

I worked in the profession within the parameters in which I was trained, but I was always looking for alternatives, because I felt that academia hadn't effectively prepared me to deal with the adversities that affect people and the daily life of the public service, which was my first job, as I couldn't afford to set up a private practice.

I came into contact with Institutional Analysis (IA) for the first time when I was a technician at the Health Workers' Education Center (CETS) at Campinas City Hall in 2004, and went to Unicamp as a special student for a course coordinated by Professor Solange L'Abbate, who later became the supervisor of this doctorate. Since then, AI has become a relevant tool for my reflections and analysis from the point of view of research, clarification of doubts, anxieties and questions about Collective Health and the way I act professionally and sentimentally in my work at SUS.

I am currently part of the CNPq Research Directory "Institutional Analysis &

---

5 MCTI/CNPq/MS-SCTIE-Decit number 10/2012 ; Bibliography number 28

Collective Health", coordinated by my advisor, in which colleagues from the Postgraduate Program in Collective Health, professors from other universities, as well as professionals from some Municipal Health Secretariats participate. Institutional Analysis and Health Practices is one of the lines of research in the Social Sciences concentration area of the postgraduate course in Collective Health at the Department of the same name in the School of Medical Sciences at Unicamp.

In my practice, I've been looking for ways to introduce an expanded oral health clinic (Campos, 2000)[29] in Primary Care[6] , from the perspective of comprehensiveness, and investigating the ways in which the Prosthesis Service, for which I am the technical manager in the Eastern District[7] , is socially instituted, as well as trying to understand the feelings of the users who utilize and use this service.

Barbara Starfield (2002)[30] considers Primary Care to be the individual's gateway to the health services system, and has the central principle of *longitudinality* as a characteristic of this level of care. This means that the professional must establish a bond with the patient/user and must maintain continuity of care, taking responsibility for it.

Although health is a constitutional right, when I look at my daily life, my activities in the Prosthesis Service, I can easily see the contradiction between this legally established achievement and the reality of the crisis experienced by users and by us SUS professionals. Among various aspects, the principle of universality, a guarantee of access for all and a duty of the state, which should allow any citizen who needs health services to be attended to and for professionals to have adequate working conditions, draws attention, but the reality is quite different.

---

6 In Brazil, the name Primary Care was adopted to counter the perspective taken by many countries and international organizations, which see Primary Care as a set of low-complexity actions dedicated to low-income populations. The designation taken by the Brazilian government therefore aims to counter the political-ideological proposal of primary care, and seeks to recover the universalist nature of the Alma Ata Declaration, reorienting the care model towards a universal and integrated health care system, which encompasses various sectors, without profit motives. (Oliveira and Pereira, 2013)
7 Campinas is administratively divided into 5 districts/regions, namely: East, North, South, Southwest and Northwest.

The complexity of the health-disease process must be widely understood in order to have an understanding of public policies, of which oral health is a part. These policies must serve and guarantee the well-being and improved quality of life of our population and this is what I have been seeking and what Collective Health has been discussing.

However, despite the technological and scientific advances in the field of oral health in Brazil, one cannot fail to mention that there have been no effective improvements in the population indicators for the most prevalent oral diseases. As stated by Kovaleski, Freitas and Botazzo (2006, p.98)[31]: "So far, it can be said that - collectively - it has failed", referring to current dentistry.

Fonsêca and Junqueira (2014 p.41 and 42)[9] , agree with Kovaleski, Freitas and Botazzo (2006)[31] and add:

Despite the increase in the number of restorative procedures and the improvement in the Brazilian population's access to medium-complexity procedures achieved with the PNSB, which has led to important epidemiological improvements, there is still a lock-in to the private sector's model of care and clinical work, with the mere reproduction of this logic in the SUS. The main points to be discussed in this regard concern the way in which dental consultations are organized, the timid presence or absence of auxiliary staff and the technologies of care that are reflected in low coverage, dental-centredness and accentuated technification. By maintaining the use of dentistry to the detriment of oral health care technologies, the grandeur of the ESF is reduced, in other words, old concepts are preserved in a new guise.

Undoubtedly, this discomfort on the part of the authors is also felt by many professionals, including myself. The lack of articulation between the degree and the field of work makes it impossible to consolidate ethical work, capable of providing care and promoting health.

Onocko Campos (2005)[32] states that people are often interested in studying issues that have marked their personal lives (as in the case of this research) and this is not necessarily a bad thing. But it has to be understood that the many variables involved in the process are not always measurable and therefore require a qualitative study rather than the more usual quantitative one involving statistics, numerical expressions of indices, coefficients and patterns, and this is how we will conduct this research.

From 2007 onwards, I became a reference for the Prosthesis Service, replacing a colleague who had been invited to be the coordinator of a Basic Health Unit. I found it very unstructured, because the laboratory that provided the service was shutting down due to technical operational problems: not only was the quality poor, but there were changes and delays in delivering the services. We spent about four months waiting for a new tender, which was won by a small laboratory from a neighboring municipality (Jaguariùna/SP). When it came time to renew the contract, the laboratory failed to meet some bureaucratic criteria, which meant it lost the tender to another laboratory in Curitiba (Paranà). Since then, the five professionals who are part of the prosthetics service in the municipality of Campinas, each in their respective district, have been experiencing serious problems, which have led to various movements[8] in search of solutions, which will be discussed later. These discussions will permeate throughout our work.

CHAPTER II: THE CLINIC OF CARE: SUBJECTIVITY AND ORALITY

I've always practiced a little differently from what I was taught in undergraduate school. Academically, we learn that first we take an anamnesis, then we fill in the clinical form, then we carry out the clinical examination and finally the treatment of the teeth and adjacent structures. The subjects that make up the dental training course provide the necessary references (Anatomy, Physiology, Pathology...) for understanding the disease, aimed at the clinical practice of dental surgeons. But the new National Curriculum Guidelines for Undergraduate Courses in the Health Area are already pointing to other needs, in order to initiate some changes in the training of professionals' hegemonic technicist practice, proposing a closer relationship with the needs of the population.

In the SUS, according to Barros and Botazzo (2011)[33], the clinical routine still remains like this, (...) "centered on treatment carried out like a production line: the dentist receives users with cavities and residual roots and releases them with restorations and sutures. Cavities are cured and teeth restored. Users go in mute and come out silent". But my career path and implications made me "different" from other dentists trained along these hegemonic lines. I liked, and still like, to talk to patients before any other activity, to listen to their stories, which often don't seem (at first) to be related to the disease being treated, to think together with them about what alternatives we might have other than those that are "standardized", protocol-based... I investigate the possibility of discussing a clinic as a powerful element in understanding the illness of that person (patient) and reflect on the possibilities of intervention beyond the limits of the diagnosis/therapy of the case, well beyond the pathological signs and symptoms. The reasons for that problem, that illness, that change, have always bothered me. I was never able to count the cavities and simply restore them.... Barros and Botazzo (2011)[33] state that traditional professional practice is not enough to carry out a clinic committed to promoting health and affirming life. Especially if we consider that health and illness don't have the same meanings for all individuals. Scliar (2007)[34] states that health and illness depend on the time, place, social class, individual values, scientific, religious and philosophical conceptions of each era, as seen in the Introduction to this work.

The reductionist paradigm of health practices, including dental practices, is being questioned, as it has shown little resolution to the real needs of the health problems of a large part of the population. There is a need to propose other ways of thinking about and doing health, affecting the way services are organized (Campos, 2003[6] ; Luz, 2009[35] ; Merhy, 2009).[36]

According to Allison, Locker and Feine (1997)[37] , since the 1980s there has been a growing debate about health-related quality of life. Various studies point to quality of life as a dynamic and complex phenomenon, which is not just the result of objective indicators, but also has subjective aspects, in other words, quality of life is linked to the subjective and objective elements of life, of the choices made by each human being.

Various changes in oral health have had an impact on the quality of life of children, adolescents, adults and the elderly. This quality of life is related to aspects of daily life that may (or may not) change due to oral diseases in terms of frequency, severity or duration, in the individual's perception of their life in general. (Bendo et al, 2014)[38] .

There has been a growing concern to investigate the repercussions of oral problems on people's quality of life, relating them to functional limitations, emotional well-being and social welfare.

Barros and Botazzo (2011)[33] state that oral health care requires prioritizing the production of subjectivity through listening to others and making diagnoses in clinical encounters that give meaning to the intervention, whatever it may be. A well conducted welcome, anamnesis and listening can be responsible for 85% of the diagnosis in the clinic, leaving 10% for the physical examination and only 5% for complementary tests.

Guattari, in his work "Chaosmosis" (1992, p.11)[39] , states that Subjectivity is plural and polyphonic and that there are at least three types of problems that urge us to broaden the definition of Subjectivity in order to overcome the classic opposition between subject and society and through this, review the model of the Unconscious, they are: ".... the irruption of subjective factors into the foreground of historical actuality, the massive development of machinic productions of subjectivity and, lastly, the recent prominence of ethological and ecological aspects relating to human subjectivity."

Still according to this author, subjective factors have always played an important role throughout history, but today they are on the verge of playing a leading role since they have been taken over by the world-wide media. He believes that "the technological machines of information and communication operate at the core of human subjectivity, not only within its memories, its Intelligence, but also its sensitivity, its affections, its unconscious phantasms." (Guattari, 1992. p.14)[39]

Finally, this author believes that in certain social contexts, subjectivity becomes individual: "a person, considered responsible for himself, positions himself in the midst of relations of alterity governed by family customs, local customs, legal laws... In other conditions, subjectivity becomes collective, which does not mean that it therefore becomes exclusively social. " (Guattari, 1992. p.19 and 20)[39] .

For this author, subjectivity is not only manufactured through the psychogenetic phases of psychoanalysis or through the unconscious, but also by social machines and the media. In other words, in general, each individual or social group conveys its own system for modeling subjectivity.

Through this logic, any event that could go unnoticed by someone can become the key to triggering a "complex rhythm" (terminology used by the author), which can modify the immediate behavior of the patient/user, opening up new fields of vision.

Simonetti (2016)[40] , defines subjectivity by relating it to the way a person experiences things in their own mind and based on feelings or opinions rather than facts.

Dental aesthetics are known to have a direct effect on an individual's self-esteem, especially if it is related to social acceptance. Damage to the front teeth due to decay, trauma, periodontal disease or severe fluorosis can affect quality of life. Physical discomfort, caused mainly by pain, and psychological discomfort, caused by the difficulty of smiling, can directly affect social interaction (Bendo et al, 2014)[38].

Aesthetic problems cause discomfort, embarrassment when smiling and relationship difficulties, with repercussions on the person's physical and emotional well-being. A *cohort* study in New Zealand, carried out by Lawrence et al, in 2008[41] , concluded that edentulous patients reported greater difficulty in pronouncing words and altered taste, as well as feeling embarrassed, irritable, having difficulty relaxing and carrying out their daily tasks.

Patients therefore need an approach that goes beyond the physical examination. Therefore, the dental surgeon's attention should be focused on other problems that are not exclusively the most prevalent oral problems, such as tooth decay and periodontal disease.

Bendo et al (2014)[38] state that all care should be based on a holistic view, i.e. looking at the individual as a whole, so that other problems can be seen and do not go unnoticed.

Guattari (1992, p.35)[39] proposes a de-centering of the question of the subject to that of subjectivity:

The subject has traditionally been conceived as the ultimate essence of individuation, as a pure, empty, pre-reflective apprehension of the world, as the focus of sensitivity and expressiveness, the unifier of states of consciousness. With subjectivity (as conceptualized by Guattari), the emphasis will instead be on the founding instance of intentionality. It is a question of taking the relationship between the subject and the object in the middle, and bringing to the foreground the instance that expresses itself. From this point on, the question of content is raised again. This participates in subjectivity, giving consistency to the ontological quality of Expression.

It is based on the assumption that people process different meanings about the various dimensions they experience, varying according to personal experience and the specific socio-historical context in which they are inserted.

In conclusion, trying to understand how people make sense of the different aspects of their realities is very complex.

This is why disregarding the patient's subjectivity and life experience implies a series of negative consequences for the professional-patient relationship, as stated by Traverso-Yépez and Morais, 2004[42] .

Thus, the practices related to the health-disease process, far from being reduced to organic and objective evidence, are closely related to the characteristics of each social context and also to the way people subjectively experience these states, as stated by Traverso-Yépez and Morais (2004, p.81)[42] :

What is interesting to realize, however, is that the daily practices of the current health system, based on the hegemonic biomedical model, continue to neglect this complexity by focusing on the disease and disregarding the value of the patient's subjective experience, as well as the permanent interdependence between the biological, psychosocial, cultural and environmental factors related to the health-disease process.

Subjectivity is considered here as the way in which people react/interact with the conditions of their lives, their histories and those of their families, as well as their class and culture. (Souza, 2004)[43]

By subjectivity we mean subjects in production, making themselves. We agree with Souza (2003, p.41)[44] :

Foucault invites us to move away from the philosophical conceptions of subject-essence towards subject-form. The historical production of subject-forms that modulate and are modulated in a permanent being. What is in the order of the production of the subject is no longer the origin and invariant, but the result of a process of modeling and remodeling, historically regulated. What exists, then, are forms of subjectification. Subjectivity is therefore multiple and plural, losing any fixity in its being.

Franco and Merhy (2013)[45] start from the premise that workers in the same team can act differently in the production of care, in different ways, even though they are under the same normative guidelines. Unlike some professionals, there are those who have **desire** (my emphasis) as a driving force, constitutive of subjectivities that make them protagonists par excellence in processes of change.

According to Deleuze and Guattari (1972)[46] desire here "is of the order of production and any production is both desiring and social". According to these authors, desire is formed in the unconscious and is a productive energy which therefore drives the construction of social reality by the subject. Thus, it cannot be guaranteed that academic training is solely responsible for the hegemonic and technical way of doing dentistry, leading some professionals to emphasize only aesthetic issues.

According to Bendo et al, (2014)[38] , there is a consensus on the importance of physical appearance in today's society. Significant changes can have an emotional impact, damaging self-esteem and affecting personal and social relationships.

It can therefore be seen that there is great complexity in the relationship between oral alterations and subjectivity. Therefore, you can't just treat the "apparent disease" or just resolve aesthetic issues.

Franco and Merhy (2013)[45] propose an approach that includes welcoming and bonding, so that the professional recognizes the subjectivity of patients. They believe that this is how live work in health takes place and can thus be seen as a micropolitics and a strategic place for change.

It can be seen that the way care is produced is effectively revealed in its micropolitics, if there is a method that is capable of verifying the dynamic and complex way in which each worker operates in their daily actions, including their subjective production in action, which produces health care and, at the same time, produces the worker themselves as a subject in the world. (Franco and Merhy, 2013, p.152)[45]

Barros and Botazzo (2011)[33] stated that listening and dialog are not gifts and that the ability to dialog is essential to the care process, requiring a willingness and technique to listen to others and their knowledge. These communication and clinical reasoning skills have a relational dimension and are therefore soft technologies (Merhy, 2002)[47] which aim to welcome the user and interfere in the evolution of their suffering, re-establishing bodily homeostasis and producing bonds.

In order to break with the nosological concepts of dentistry that have been guiding undergraduate courses, hegemonically centered on teeth and surgery as the *priority* for diagnosis and therapy, Barros and Botazzo (2011)[33] suggest using other theoretical-methodological references, such as that of oral health.

Orality is understood as an expression of the social work carried out by the human mouth, thus showing that the mouth is not isolated, but is part of a body, which is the result of biological, psychic and affective factors. This term establishes the relationship between the oral cavity and its articulation with people's lives, which goes far beyond the functions attributed to the mouth and its organs, such as language and chewing.

All mammals, from a biological point of view, have an organ for feeding, the mouth, with anatomical structures such as the tongue, teeth, glands, bones, muscles, among others, but only the human species have other functions besides feeding (chewing): eroticism and language. (Botazzo, 2000[48] . 2008[49] . 2013)[50]

The term "bucality" broadens the concept of "mouth", which is generally seen only as an organ for speech and feeding. This terminology is an alternative for a new understanding of the mouth and oral health, when we try to bring it into the clinic.

It is from an understanding of health as a state of unstable equilibrium determined socially and subjectively by *homo sapiens*, from the re-signification of the social functions of the mouth, from the understanding of oral and dental illness and from the constitution of the clinical case in the anamnesis that another position for the clinic will be established. Barros and Botazzo (2011, p.4347)[33].

For this reason, studying teeth and the mouth only as functional organs is not enough to explain the complex web of desires, pleasures and feelings that are involved with this organ. Botazzo states that, in order to do this, it is necessary to see the mouth in movement with the world and it was in this sense that the author developed this concept of bucality, in order to broaden the understanding of the complexity that exists in this territory, called the human mouth.

(...) despite the fact that it is a region made up of viscera (muscles, tongue, glands, teeth, mucous membranes), and despite the fact that each one of them has its own physiology, the work they do expresses functional synergy; separately they can do nothing. Unlike other organs or regions of the body, the functions of the human mouth are socially defined. Any one of its functions expresses a link with culture and the psyche. This is obvious. The permissions or ethical authorizations for such uses are therefore variable historically and according to models of sociability specific to each society and at a given moment in its organization. We can speak of a psychogenesis and a socio-genesis of the mouth. For this reason alone, the human mouth is strongly linked to the civilizing process. (Botazzo, 2011[51] , p.2 and 3)

It is therefore possible to find other senses and meanings that go beyond the functions privileged in anatomy and physiology manuals (Botazzo, 2000[48] , 2008[49] , 2013[50]), as Cartesian science alone is not capable of understanding all the senses of the mouth. Human sciences disciplines such as sociology, psychology, philosophy and others are necessary to train a professional who will be dealing with human beings and not just isolated organs outside the body.

Oral diseases can affect people's eating, sleeping, speech, communication, oral health, social interaction and self-esteem, causing difficulties in their daily activities and impairing their quality of life.

Botazzo (2013, p. 9)[50] also states that the mouth is an organ that stands out from all the others in the human body, since it is through it that we carry out social activities and, furthermore, the human mouth "plays an unparalleled role in the formation of the psyche (or subjectivity), as well as the individual's identity, and is a relevant part of the bodily structures linked to desire". According to this author:

Except for the sucking ability with which mammalian babies are structurally endowed - therefore innate - and which guarantees their survival in a specific way on the evolutionary scale, from then on, all the oral manifestations of the human mammal will bear the **mark of** the **social,** whether in feeding, communication, affectivity, love relationships and so many other activities that men (women, children, adults or old people) do with the oral cavity as a support. (Bold by the author)

The same author also refers to the mouth we're talking about as the social mouth, the mouth that speaks, moans, laughs and sings. The mouth that communicates with the world. The entrance ostium to the world of the body. It speaks of a mouth full of sociological and psychological aspects and a producer of subjectivities. A concrete mouth, scrutinized and controlled, but misunderstood. In the mouths of the people, the "pierced tooth", for the group that insists on wearing white, the demineralization of the enamel promoted by the acid attack resulting from the bacterial metabolism of the sugars ingested in the diet. (Botazzo, 2000[48] ; Kovaleski, 2004).[52]

Agreeing with Botazzo, Souza, in 2004[43] , at the exhibition of the III State Conference on Oral Health in Rio Grande do Norte, stated that a clinic that takes the mouth as a fragmented organ and detached from the body becomes a "de-humanized" mouth, because the civilizational and psychic aspects have been disregarded[9] and adds to the discussion the "violence of the naturalization of dental loss, which is a symbol of the social exclusion of many Brazilians who, by exposing their dental loss, are also exposing their cultural, social, economic, emotional and political losses, among others. "

Kovaleski, Freitas and Botazzo (2006, p.102)[31] conclude that:

Orality, as well as the set of debates it gives rise to, constitutes a field, until now theoretical, that represents the possibility of change, the negation of this

---

9 Oral presentation by the author at the III State Health Conference in Rio Grande do Norte, 2004.

alienated, isolated and discriminated dentistry and mouth, for another, more autonomous, more collective and more politicized.

Recognizing the importance of and valuing the user's ideas and beliefs, as well as their subjective dimension and their mouth, means believing that in the user-professional relationship there is ethical respect and acceptance of the knowledge/knowledge of the "other".

In fact, this relationship is almost always based on the belief that only the health professional, and not the patient themselves, knows about their state of health or illness. Communication between them tends to be unsatisfactory, both because of the time constraints and consequent lack of availability that most professionals face because they have to juggle different activities, and because they are insufficiently prepared to listen to and talk to the patient. Another aspect that hampers communication is the professional's use of technical language, which is often difficult to understand by the lay user and the poorly educated (Traverso-Yépez and Morais, 2004)[42].

We understand that communication is the raw material of dialog and dialog is not a small thing; on the contrary, it means having the willingness to understand/accept different points of view that can come together or clash, merge or complement each other. "These are interests, needs, knowledge, cultural codes, institutional rituals, scientific ingredients and others from the social field. Dialogue allows even contradictory knowledge to circulate, because "they are reserved for otherness in interaction, in contact, in connection." (Martines and Machado, 2010, p. 331 and 332)[53]

These same authors carried out a bibliographic review for a doctoral project which aimed to carry out a theoretical reflection in which there was a connection between the production of care and subjectivity, in order to understand the ideas developed to support this connection. Through the website www.usp.br/sibi, they accessed the "Dedalus - global online catalog", and then selected the words: subjectivity and care. They found 26 records, of which only two were not analyzed.

Martines and Machado (2010)[53] observed that some authors referred to the notion of subjectivity as part of a dimension

This is necessary to make up a vision of the integrality of the human being. Carrying out technical care where the plane of technicality prevails is pushing aside other planes, including that of subjectivity. Thus, the form of treatment focused on the disease, on functional alterations and not on the subject is doomed to failure.

They then proposed that at least collecting a good clinical history is important in order to create spaces in which we can talk about the subject's relationships with their family, work, affective dimensions, culture, leisure, among other aspects that have the same importance as their sleep pattern, blood pressure, whether they have undergone surgery, where they were born, their family background, whether they smoke, among others. They understood that subjectivity refers to the possibilities of existence, stories and experiences; it incorporates choices and social characteristics. This is how we "collected" the interviews for this research, which were then "transformed" into pathographies[10] .

In agreement with the authors cited above, Traverso-Yépez and

Morais (2004)[42] also believes that the notion of subjectivity extends to all those involved in the production of care and this includes users and workers.

Thus, the production of care refers to the day-to-day running of services, exactly as in the case of this thesis, and refers to the events, situations, manifestations and details that are part of every day life.

According to Martines and Machado (2010, p.329)[53] :

In a first conception, it can be said that **care** is everything that comes together in the form of actions or interventions that help to generate, organize or (re)establish hope, autonomy, freedom of choice, human relationships and the meaning of life.

Therefore, it is proposed that there should be care for users, in addition to the

---

10 Pathographies: Terminology that refers to the way subjects understand their illness throughout their history. This will be discussed in more depth in the Methodology section.

creation of a bond, the extended clinic, anamnesis and qualified listening, valuing oral health and subjectivity.

Meetings between the subjects and the professionals who will assist them.

"Encounter" here doesn't just refer to the word described in the Aurélio Dictionary (it refers to a face-to-face position with a person or thing, or to a collision of two bodies), but as stated by Mendes, Pezzato and Sacardo (2016, p.1738)[54] :

(...) the encounter is equivalent to the vital moment for the formation and creation of anything or event: it is from the meeting of two atoms that matter emerges; from the meeting between managers, professionals and users that health action emerges; from the meeting of social sectors that Inter-sectoral projects emerge; from the meeting between subjects and the territory where they build their processes of territoriality. Every "good encounter" with other bodies, to paraphrase Deleuze in his reading of Spinoza, provokes the generation of power.

According to Franco and Merhy (2013)[45] the production of subjectivity takes place through "affective factors", i.e. events that have an impact on individuals and their way of understanding the world. In our understanding, when there are "encounters", i.e. relational processes that are driven by the freedom immanent in Live Work, in act, there are relations/connections between many workers and users. In other words, "encounters" take place.

Finally, we believe that respecting the other person's subjectivity is to allow a horizontal encounter to be established, providing opportunities for care and positive achievements for both sides, i.e. in our case, the edentulous patient and the professional.

Understanding the oral health clinic beyond clinical dental care (in this case, making prostheses), the idea of innovating in the production of care in this service went far beyond carrying out an analysis of the concrete working conditions. We began to use and experiment with different tools proposed by the multicentre project (Botazzo, 2012)[28] which we talked about at the beginning of this paper: anamnesis, consultation, organization and discussions with the various people involved in the services.

It's important to note that the anamnesis used here is not similar to the one usually practiced. As qualified listening, this step in the clinical work is of the utmost importance in order to make the individual welcome, process the bond and allow the patient to talk about their discomfort, their clinical condition, their symptoms, their expectations, their life. The professional should conduct the conversation in an atmosphere of cordiality, allowing the patient to express themselves freely and interrupting with questions or observations in order to allow or facilitate the deposit of subjective material. (Botazzo, Technical Report, 2015, p. 15)[55]

Experiencing these innovations made it possible to notice and be sensitive to issues that had previously gone unnoticed. Qualified listening enabled us to discern the singularities of individuals, their mouths and subjectivities. Many users who came to the service didn't necessarily just need dentures. Many had other needs, such as restorations, extractions, periodontal treatment, among others, and sometimes demands were detected that didn't even indicate a prosthesis, or even a dental clinic, as we can see in the researcher's diary:

Today I saw a lady who had a stroke and was left with several sequelae. She can no longer walk, hardly moves her arms and has great difficulty speaking. She was accompanied by her daughter who told me that she had "had" her teeth pulled out because they were ugly and damaged... I had to take a deep breath as I listened to her story, and an even deeper one as I explained that rehabilitating this lady with two total prostheses was not the solution; on the contrary, it would be an additional inconvenience (...). At the end of the conversation, the lady, with a lot of effort, gave a big smile and thanked me. In fact, this was not her wish but her daughter's. (Diary of 11/10/2013)

At another time in my life, I might have received this lady and her daughter and proceeded to shape the alveolar ridges ("edentulous gingival margins") and then make the prostheses ("dentures"), but the innovation in care, the encounter, the respect for the subjectivity and the mouth of that lady made me realize how much the difficulty of adapting, chewing and speaking would be compromised if the dentures her daughter wanted were made. Not to mention the fact that it was only her daughter's wish, as she believed she was "doing the best for her mother" ...

Finally, we agree with Souza (2004, p.2)[43] when he states that "users who bring their complaints to the health service need to be understood as subjects who also produce themselves in illness" and, therefore, comprehensive care requires changes in the work process.

CHAPTER III: EDENTULISM IN CHILDHOOD, ADULTHOOD AND OLD AGE

On one occasion, I saw a very nervous mother who came to the office and reported that her 10-year-old son no longer wanted to go to school. I asked the mother to come in, sit down and we started talking. She told me that her son's grades had been falling for some time, there had been complaints from the teacher that the child was aggressive and, finally, a depressive process had set in, to the point where he didn't even want to play anymore. The guidance counselor was called in and after some time the problem was discovered: he was being bullied. A hit-and-run accident (trauma) had caused his upper central incisors to become avulsed and now his classmates at school were calling him "banguelo" and "toothless".

When you're 6 or 7 years old and the first deciduous teeth undergo risolysis (physiological resorption of the roots), family members and the children themselves usually celebrate and play various games, maintaining the specific culture that involves joy and magic, but when you're 10, and the teeth are already permanent, there's no more fun or reason to be happy, quite the opposite...

I knew the service's protocol well and making prostheses for children wasn't part of it. But I had to do something, because the child's subjectivity and oral health were affected.

In the Health Services, the epidemiological reference to guide program proposals is always based on population information, produced from the organization and manipulation of data under a logic of inductive inference of patients in the population, established by statistical significance (Souza, 2003)[44]. Thus, according to this reasoning, everything on the edge of the curve considered normal would be left out of the statistics and, therefore, out of the priorities for care and assistance. This has been the main way in which epidemiological knowledge has been used to define health actions, translated into population diagnoses.

These types of data are undoubtedly important guidelines for planning health policies and programs. They are valuable tools for resource management and evaluations, but they become "rigid" if they are not used with caution, as they fail to take into account particularities and singularities and end up valuing numerical data more than people. We agree that epidemiological information is extremely important for services, but we would like to draw attention to other individual needs that don't always appear because they don't fall within the parameters of statistical normality. For example, the repercussions of illness, as in the case of this child.

In Campinas, the epidemiological data, especially in the eastern district where I live, points to a large number of elderly people and, not only that, there was a movement on the part of the city's Council for the Elderly for the prosthetics project to be geared towards them. For this reason, our protocol only included the elderly in prosthetic rehabilitation treatments.

In this child's case, the illness was a fact. There was no pain, no damaged teeth, but the child was sad, very upset about the situation and his mother believed that we could treat him, perhaps make a prosthesis? So she came to see us. She gave us a try, because she had heard that we were attentive enough to look for alternatives...

We believe that the clinic of welcoming, of qualified listening, of dialog, of looking beyond the disease, can bring valuable reflections to the impasses we often face. Disregarding the patient's subjectivity, oral health and lived experience implies a series of serious consequences for the outcome(s) of the treatment(s).

Merhy (1994)[56] draws attention to the current model in public health, which is liberal-privatist, and which ends up provoking an attitude on the part of the workers, "led by the doctor-centered style", which treats the user in an impersonal, objectifying and uncommitted way. The main consequence of the distancing observed in the relationship between professional and patient is the lack of commitment on the part of the patient to the proposed/"imposed" treatment and on the part of the doctor to the cure/solution of the problem.

The moment a child came to me without permanent upper front teeth, I felt obliged to take some non-protocol action. This was because a referral for implants was out of the question, as there was a need to wait for facial bone growth to finish. Immediate action was needed to resolve (or at least alleviate) the situation.

There was a concern with social reintegration, with the quality of life of the child who had lost his teeth in the accident... The humanization of the professional-patient relationship, based on the development of empathy and participation, had to be a priority at this point, because according to Merhy (1997)[57] and Mendes (1999)[58] , it's not enough to worry about the organizational procedures of institutions if we don't change the way we relate to our main object of work: the life and suffering of the user.

Trave rso-Yépez and Morais (2004, p.82)[42] state that "the importance of political decision-making bodies is not denied, but the role of the professional in defining the type of relationship established with the user in consulting rooms, or wherever health action is carried out, should be emphasized". A humanized and horizontal approach must always prevail.

We then proposed making an "*appliance*" with the teeth in acrylic resin to replace those lost in the trauma/car accident and we are monitoring it periodically, with the piece being replaced once a year until the facial bone growth is complete, and then we will send it to the implant service of universities or partner institutions of the SUS, since we don't have this specialty in Campinas.

Once I had seen the joy and transformation that had taken place in the child's smile and life, and thinking about the huge number of people who "knocked on my door" looking for solutions to their problems, their absences and partial or total loss of teeth that had been causing them inconvenience, difficulties and even illness, I decided to take a stand and fight for the protocol to be extended beyond just treatment for the elderly. I needed to find a way out of the confinement of the service.

So, in a move to establish ourselves, we managed to prepare some audiovisual material and schedule a meeting at the Eastern District headquarters with the technical supporter and a representative from each of the 10 Basic Health Units that referred patients to us. It wasn't difficult to make everyone aware of the problem of edentulism that was alarming us. There were many more people with missing teeth and related problems than there were elderly people on the waiting lists.

In fact, the classic epidemiological studies carried out in dentistry have still provided information pointing to caries and gingivitis as the most prevalent diseases. However, the social conditions of individuals, as well as the hegemonic practice of oral health professionals, contribute significantly to the issues surrounding tooth loss. The Projeto Saùde Bucal (SB) Brasil 2010 (BRASIL, 2011)[59] in its final considerations, states that edentulism continues to be a serious problem in our country, especially among the elderly, but that the need for some kind of prosthesis begins to emerge very early, from the age group of 15 to 19 years old.

This data was confirmed by Lewandowski and Bós

(2014)[60] , in a study that looked at the use and need for dentures in the elderly. They found that edentulism in the elderly can reach 81.6% in the over 60s. This affects chewing and digestion, as well as taste, speech and aesthetics. They also assessed that an individual who has all his teeth has a chewing capacity of 100%, but when he loses a tooth, this capacity drops to 70% and can reach 25%, even with the use of prostheses.

The same authors also stated that the prevalence of edentulous elderly people in Brazil exceeds the findings of other countries, such as China, for example, which is 4.4%, or India, which is 15%, or France, which is 16.3%.

In Brazil, the first data on oral health conditions was presented in an epidemiological survey carried out in 1986 (Brasil, 1988)[61] which showed the result of a dental practice characterized by mass extractions, increasing the need for rehabilitation with dental prostheses. According to Pinto, (1988)[62] , this situation was due to the great complexity of social, economic and biological factors, with a strong influence from the mutilating curative model offered by dental services at the time. It was an exclusionary and welfare-oriented practice.

Also according to the SB Brasil 2010 criteria (Brasil, 2011)[59] , our most recent report on the oral health conditions of the population, the percentage of 68.8% of people in need of oral prostheses in the 35-44 age group is worrying, especially when we consider that Brazil is the country with the largest absolute number of dentists and that these are distributed unevenly across the country's regions. Brazil is home to 19% of the world's dentists. The data comes from the book "Perfil Atual e Tendência do Cirurgiao-Dentista Brasileiro", which was launched at the 28th Ciosp (International Dental Congress of São Paulo), held at Anhembi, São Paulo, in 2016. According to Morita (2016)[63], one of the authors of the book, Brazil is the country with the largest number of dental professionals in the world in absolute numbers: there are 219,575 professionals registered with the Federal Council of Dentistry (CFO), but this number has not contributed to minimizing the problem of edentulism.

That's why we now welcome the elderly, young people, adults and children without distinction for prostheses. There's still a lot to be worked out, as we'll discuss and analyze in the course of this research, but it was a huge step forward! An analyzer[11] that generated an instituting movement, the construction of a new practice, and which culminated in expanding users' access to the service.

Franco and Merhy (2013, p.68)[45] argue that:

The construction of a solidary future for the SUS presupposes the existence of devices capable of organizing the construction of new knowledge and practices that give new meaning to health work and, above all, to **care** (my emphasis). The agency of desires capable of operating in the construction of a new SUS presupposes confronting the territories that currently structure health services and, above all, breaking with their capitalist and capitalist becoming.

---

11 *The term "Analyzer" will be discussed in the next chapter.*

CHAPTER IV: ANALYZERS

Analyzers are defined by L'Abbate (2012, p.200)[64] as "facts and situations that arise unexpectedly, or not, in the intervention process and that allow us to identify contradictory and hidden aspects of the group or organization in which the participants are inserted". In other words, the analyzer would have the effect of revealing something that had remained hidden, disorganizing what had been organized and giving a different meaning/path to a given situation.

We believe that the event that happened to the child (reported in the previous chapter) was a powerful analyzer of one of the problems that remained "hidden" in the Prosthesis Service. Analyzers can also emerge in research situations, and not just in interventions, as we will see in various situations throughout this thesis.

L'Abbate (2004, p.82)[65] , also states:

The concept of analyzer and its application constitute a true epistemological inversion, since they produce a union between analysis and the phenomenon that engenders it, thus causing an inversion of the relationship between the real object and the object of knowledge, to the extent that they are no longer considered as separate entities.

According to Lourau (2014, p.303)[22] analyzer is everything that "allows us to reveal the structure of the organization, to provoke it, to force it to speak. Institutional provocation, institutional *acting out,* because they refer to psychosociological reference systems (emotional provocation), or psychoanalytical (*acting out)*".

Dobies and L'Abbate (2016, p.128)[66] state that the analyzer is one of the main concepts of Institutional Analysis and "was initially used by chemists and physicists as a natural or constructed element capable of breaking down material reality into its component elements for experimentation and analysis".

Lapassade (1979)[67] reports that the opposition between analyzers and analysts functions as a revealer, as an analyzer of our society and its institutions. And indeed, the episode of that child without his front permanent teeth worked as an analyzer to open my eyes to the vehement need to transform the protocol.

Hess and Savoye (1993, p.105)[68] point out that "by analyzer, we mean the elements which, through the contradictions of various kinds that they introduce, make it possible to enunciate the determinations of the situation".

And that's exactly what we discovered in that child's situation. There was a gap between management (protocols), the care we provided and the need for places for treatment and/or prosthetic replacement felt by the users, and this diminished our ability to value the transformative potential of our practices.

In Collective Health, dental surgeons are invited to rethink their practice and play new roles within dentistry. Professionals have a responsibility to advocate for healthy public policies and to help people empower themselves in their quest for quality of life (Sheiham and Moyses, 2000).[69]

Thus, as stated by Aerts, Abegg and Cesa (2004)[70] , the dental surgeon has an important role to play in guiding people to identify beliefs that are harmful to health; in encouraging children and adults to have their mouths examined to detect problems and in advising where to seek help; as well as training community agents and assistants; continuing education for other professionals; collective educational actions in schools, local councils, associations related to lifestyle, fluoride use, guidance, among others. In fact, our role as health educators is very broad and goes beyond guidance to meet/seek the autonomy of users.

Also according to these authors, health-promoting dental services involve the presence of professionals with a broad view of the health-disease process, capable of understanding people, taking into account the various aspects of their lives, and not just a set of signs and symptoms restricted to the oral cavity.

It can be said that interest in the social sciences in Brazil began in the late 1960s and early 1970s, with the realization of the importance of social determinants in the health-disease process. Since then, attempts have been made to reconstruct explanatory models aimed at comprehensive patient care and the integration of biological, psychological and social knowledge in understanding the disease(s).

Almeida et al (2010)[71] state that oral health is not just the result of dental practice, but of social constructions carried out consciously by all individuals in each particular situation and, being a social process, each situation is unique, singular and historical, It cannot be mechanically replicated or reproduced in any other concrete situation, since the elements and dimensions of each of these processes present contradictions, generate conflicts and are marked by negotiations that are specific to them.

Many situations speak for themselves and this child's story was no different, allowing me to reflect on the object of my daily life; allowing me to understand and learn that absolutely real and new cases occur every day and that we need to look at them creatively. The inclusion of oral health in the Family Health strategy, through financial incentives (including for prostheses) represented the possibility of creating spaces for practices and relationships to be built in order to reorient our own work, although the essence of this program has not yet reached all professionals, teams, municipalities...

Ferreira et al (2006)[72] , believe that in the social spaces of dental services, which focus on care, a new perspective based on social representations is favored, going beyond the normative sphere. This view expresses the subjectivity of reality, rather than restricting itself to technical issues.

For these authors (p.213)[72] oral health care has merited important considerations in the context of health policies, because the loss of teeth has various "psychosocial implications that lead to the manifestation of different behaviors, such as intimidation and shyness, due to biological, physical and emotional changes", exactly as happened in the case of the child.

As reported in the previous chapter, by welcoming that mother, listening to her, giving her the necessary attention and looking for ways to help and solve her problem, we were paying attention to an important analyzer. In addition, we were giving them the autonomy to seek out the resources needed to strengthen actions (social control), which is also the responsibility of health professionals and is one of the most important conditions for promoting the oral health of the population, with a view to integrating the traditional approach. The community is considered a fundamental resource for building oral health. In this sense, the active involvement of the population in issues they know like no one else is essential, acting in decision-making, planning and implementing actions, as well as monitoring the resources used.

Thinking about the concepts of Collective Health and linking them to oral health doesn't just mean developing actions and procedures in social spaces, homes and health units, such as health and epidemiological surveillance, diagnosis, prevention and treatment of plaque diseases, fluoride therapy, early diagnosis of oral cancer and diseases with oral manifestations, as well as educational activities which are of great importance. But to carry out the Extended Clinic, comprehensive care! Thus, the notion of Primary Care presupposes health units and workers in charge of actions that are no less complex than those considered Medium and High complexity. They are certainly less technologically dense, but the management of various health problems does not constitute a set of low-complexity technologies, as was perceived in the case of the child.

CHAPTER V: CONTEXTUALIZING AND SITUATING THE RESEARCH THE NATIONAL ORAL HEALTH POLICY (PNSB)

The National Oral Health Policy (PNSB), instituted in 2004, had the fundamental objective of inducing the reorganization of Primary Care in relation to Oral Health actions and, to this end, included in its strategy the induction of policies anchored in the transfer of funds to fund and implement its guidelines in Brazilian municipalities (Martino, 2011)[73] . It also pointed out guidelines for reorganizing actions and reorienting the country's oral health care model, with the concept of care as its central axis, proposing assumptions for expanding and qualifying oral health care from the perspective of comprehensive care. These include: qualification of primary care, guaranteeing quality and resolubility; primary care articulated with the network of services; integrality of actions, articulating the individual and the collective, promotion and prevention, treatment and recovery of the population in question.

The PNSB, better known as Smiling Brazil, was approved by the National Health Councils, State and Municipal Secretariats and became part of the National Health Plan, instituted by Ministerial Order 2.607, of 10/12/2004 (Brasil, 2004)[12] . This program was officially presented as an expression of a sub-sectoral policy, embodied in the document Diretrizes da Politica Nacional de Saùde Bucal (Guidelines for the National Oral Health Policy), defined within the framework of the 2003-2006 government, with financial investments never before made in Brazilian oral health (Frazâo and Narvai, 2009)[14] .

The PNSB lays down rules for the transfer of funds. This concerns the creation of ESBs linked to the Family Health Strategy and the creation of Dental Specialty Centers (CEO), as well as the introduction of the Regional Dental Prosthesis Laboratories (LRPD), which is relevant to this research and will be discussed during the course of this work (Brasil, 2006)[11] .

The implementation of Dental Specialty Centers (DSC), the possibility of making prostheses, as well as the improvement of existing services, universalizing access and promoting protection and prevention, as well as treatment and rehabilitation, with the consequent maintenance of integral health, should be a reality for the entire population, since there has long been talk of dentistry's social debt to the Brazilian population (Araùjo and Zilbovicius, 2004)[74] .

However, despite this recommended policy, a study conducted in the country by Ferreira et al (2006)[72], points out that the main complaints reported by SUS users are the need for more vacancies and the lack of rehabilitative treatment (prostheses) in the dental service, as found in this thesis.

The SUS should be seen as a great possibility for redeeming this debt, and it is undoubtedly making progress, as demonstrated by the PNSB, insofar as it advocates a new model of intervention, with a clinic that is more in tune with the needs of the public system. However, unlike the technicist and biologicist model, centered on procedures, we see difficulties in our daily lives that are shared by other authors/researchers, as we will list below.

Until recently, there weren't many studies associating tooth loss with the impact on people's lives, but in the last decade there has been a significant increase in interest in these issues, as well as a desire to quantify the problems generated in individuals with partial or total edentulism.

If we think that mass tooth extraction began in the 1930s as a practical and economical solution to solve the problems associated with people's teeth, especially in the low-income social class, we will agree with Guimarâes and Marcos (1996)[75] who, after examining 414 patients living in Belo Horizonte, observed that practically 50% of the extracted elements in this social class were recoverable. In the same study, the authors concluded that the number of lost teeth increased with age, and was 2.5 times higher in the low-income social class, which shows that social risk is a determining factor in tooth loss.

Silva, Magalhâes and Ferreira (2010)[76] also concluded that functional and psychological aspects, trauma and rejection in interpersonal relationships as a result of missing teeth are elements pointed out and faced in the daily lives of toothless people. The research also showed that the causes of tooth loss were associated with a lack of knowledge, difficulty in accessing services and solutions to pain. Finally, they found that "total tooth loss has a strong impact on people's lives and implies negative consequences such as shame, difficulty eating, damage to personal relationships and a feeling of 'incompleteness'".

Based on the narratives of residents of a poor community in the Northeast of Brazil, Moreira, Nations and Alves (2007 p.1388)[77] concluded that the condition of oral health/disease is a reflection of family income, individual income, access to services and social communication networks. In addition, they stressed that the challenge of adequate and humanized access to oral health services involves the elitist dimension of dental treatment, since "...the association between poverty, poor oral health and difficulty in accessing the service leads the population to a penalizing condition that increases social inequalities through the reduction of opportunities for advancement in life..."

Souza (2011, p.221)[78] considered that for the toothless population, "dental loss reflects only part of the lost or completely denied opportunities to take in the world and life".

He also said that the naturalization of tooth loss produces the aesthetic of the "banguela", visualized in the lower classes who are outside the productive system, and therefore excluded from the possibility of consumption, including health goods.

Vargas and Paixâo (2005)[79] observed that psychosocial and functional problems reported by toothless people interfere with quality of life and that the number of missing teeth in the adult Brazilian population is directly related to the need to use prostheses and the lack of access to this service.

Goffman (1988)[80] stated that when an individual has a different trait or characteristic, or a physical deformity, they can be rejected. In this case, they have a stigma and are incapable of social acceptance. This is how the theory of the relationship between appearance and stigma was formed. It is believed that people measure others by their appearance and that the face is the most differentiated part of the body. Therefore, in Western culture, missing teeth (especially front teeth) are a facial disfigurement that constitutes a stigma.

Botazzo, in 2000[48], stated that oral health has been understood as the ability of the mouth to be a mouth, that is, to perform the functions for which it is anatomically suited without limitation or impairment. But when we look at the pathographies (which will be described later), we see that the population has been suffering for many years because of tooth loss and the problems generated by this loss, in other words, oral health is shaken.

According to the Journal of the Federal Council of Dentistry No. 103 (Apr-May-Jun 2012)[81] previous governments have recognized and prioritized oral health, understanding the need to restore the dignity of the population by giving them back the right to smile and, above all, to have their chewing functions back through dental prostheses. Thus, through the Brasil Sorridente Program, R$ 6.3 million would be allocated in resources for the implementation of 908 Oral Health Teams; R$ 16.2 million for the opening of new Regional Dental Prosthesis Laboratories; and R$ 132 million a year in readjustment of the financial incentives for the implementation and costing of Dental Specialty Centers, with a variation between 25% and 50% readjustment for

the cost of maintenance and the purchase of materials needed for operation. This measure provided for in ordinances 1.109 and 1.110 was published in the Official Gazette of the Union on May 29, 2012 and would benefit 249 municipalities in 21 states plus the Federal District, including Campinas/SP, which is the site of our research.

But do the municipalities have enough capacity to produce policies to encourage these transfers? Would the funds be used in a coherent/legitimate way by the managers? Are local and municipal councils empowered enough to carry out social control? These issues were not the subject of this thesis, but the question remains: would decentralization of the implementation of municipal decision-making autonomy in relation to federal policies and sub-national coordination mechanisms have the potential to contribute to the implementation and qualification of oral health services at local level, specifically in the area of prosthetics, in the municipality of Campinas/SP, which is the site of this study?

We would like to see if the supply to the population of Campinas is in line with demand. Has all the political and financial investment by the Ministry of Health had repercussions for those who need this service? Is this new approach in the dental clinic of rehabilitating partially and totally edentulous patients, with a view to reintegrating them into society and restoring their self-esteem, really a possibility? Has such an investment really had an impact on the users who benefit from the service? What do they think about it? Is it possible to verify this in reports and "Pathographic Stories" (Souza, 2011)[78]? Are we succeeding in producing care or are we just trying to put into practice the guidelines that are so well elucidated in a law that is (im)possible to implement?

These are the main questions that this research aims to address.

Still contextualizing and situating the research

The Municipality of Campinas and the SUS Prosthesis Service:

Campinas has around 1,100,000 inhabitants, among whom are minorities who concentrate income and wealth, with a consumption pattern similar to that of the United States and wealthy European countries. The newspaper "Folha de Sao Paulo", of 01/07/2015[82], states that the metropolitan region is second in the "ranking" of the country's Human Development Index (HDI), but despite this, it still has many inhabitants who live in environments of intense poverty and violence.

It is estimated that around 70% of this population is SUS dependent, with no financial resources or health plans to access care/treatment for the diseases and illnesses that affect them. (Campinas, 2001 - the city council's website only has data up to this year)[83] .

L'Abbate (2010)[84] , in reviewing the history of the implementation of public health care in Campinas, reports that until the 1970s, the public service consisted of a few Health Centers and Posts run by the State and Municipal Secretariats, an Emergency Room (today the Dr. Màrio Gatti Municipal Hospital), a Municipal Hospital and INAMPS outpatient clinics. In 1977 and 1978, 16 more health centers were set up, in addition to the four that already existed.

It was only in 1983 that a process of integration between the various services began. In January 1989, Gastâo Wagner de Sousa Campos, a professor at the Department of Preventive and Social Medicine, now the Department of Collective Health at Unicamp's Faculty of Medical Sciences, took over the Municipal Health Department for the first time and proposed discussing issues relating to the situation and organization of services. At the time, the basic network consisted of 38 Municipal Health Centers, 5 Health Centers and a Mental Health Outpatient Clinic, as well as 4 PUC Campinas Health Centers.

It is worth noting that the city's Health Department in the 1980s was innovative in incorporating auxiliary staff, creating modular spaces for dental care and expanding population coverage (Manfredini, 200885, L'Abbate, 2010).[84]

Today, the health network is made up of different types of units with different responsibilities. There are 63 Basic Health Units, five (5) large hospitals (Mario Gatti, Campo Grande, Ouro Verde, Sâo José and Anchieta), regionalized Health Surveillance Units, the SAMU, three specialty clinics, 13 Psychosocial Care Centres - CAPS, one (1) Rehabilitation Centre, one (1) Workers' Health Reference Centre, one (1) Reference Center for the STD/AIDS Program, one (1) Zoonosis Surveillance Unit, one (1) Lactation Center, two (2) Dental Specialty Centers, three (3) Home Care Services (SAD), 14 Social Centers, two (2) Pharmacies and one (1) Botica, the CEASA Outpatient Clinic, among others. (www.campinas.sp.gov.br)[83]

It's worth noting here that the two Dental Specialty Centers, one in the southwest region and the other in the northwest region, include the Prosthesis Services of their respective districts. The other three services, in the other regions, as in our case, in the eastern region, are inside Basic Units, but operate as a specialty.

In January 2001, Mayor Antônio da Costa Santos, or "Toninho do PT", took over the municipal administration and reappointed Gastâo Wagner de Sousa Campos as municipal health secretary. Thus, the Paidéia Family Health Project was launched. This proposed care model was based on the Family

Health Program with modifications and new emphases.

The Paidéia Project (Campos, 2000)[29] has as its guidelines the creation of bonds, prioritization of risks and socio-epidemiological vulnerability, as well as the logic of the Extended Clinic, which aims to produce health by relieving symptoms and caring for people, preventing illnesses, curing and rehabilitating patients and their families. The project also advocates increased autonomy and expands the capacity for self-care, as well as the way of analyzing the health-disease process and intervening in it.

In April, still in 2001, the Paidéia Oral Health Seminar was held, with representatives from the central and district levels and service directors. The product of the Seminar was a document that would serve as the basis for the oral health policy of the 2001-2004 administration and which assumed that the network would be organized based on the interests of the population and not just the particular interests of the professionals (Manfredini, 2008)[85] .

In 2004, the Dental Prosthesis project was set up in the municipality in response to the demands of the Council for the Elderly. There was no significant investment as only five (5) professionals from other services were sent to work 20 hours a week per region (district), with the aim of making total and social prostheses[12] for the Basic Units in each of the city's district regions, namely: North, South, East, Northwest and Southwest.

Although the clinical phase of the installation of elementary dental prostheses belongs to Primary Care, the services work as referrals (Secondary Care) for the units in their respective regions. Specifically in the Eastern District, which is the site of this research, there are 10 units that refer users to a single professional (in this case the researcher) and, as a result, the "waiting lists" are enormous, and it can take five years for a user to be called in for a dental prosthesis.

According to Stake (2011, p.25)[86] , many people who conduct qualitative research want to improve the way services work. "Empathy and advocacy are

---

12 *Social prostheses or popularly known as "pererecas", are temporary prostheses, usually made to partially rehabilitate individuals without anterior teeth.*

and should be part of the researcher's lifestyle. However, focusing on doing good can interfere with understanding how things work and, ultimately, can minimize improvements by framing the work too simply." We don't want this to interfere with our understanding, and for this reason we believe that presenting some figures on the service's assistance can help us in our reflections and interpretations.

This research is in fact qualitative and aims to understand the phenomena that involve the subjectivity/mouth of edentulous patients and their relationship with the prosthesis service, since we are trying to understand meanings and not quantities, but we will provide some numerical data just to give visibility to the context in which the prosthesis service is inserted.

TABLE 1: RATIO OF HEALTH CENTERS TO THE NUMBER OF PEOPLE IN THEIR POPULATION

Health Centers belonging to the Eastern District	Average Population in number of inhabitants by region (Data provided by the Coordinators of the respective Health Units)
Costa e Silva	33.000
Taquaral	45.000
Center	70.000
Sâo Quirino	28.100
Conceiçao	25.000
Carlos Gomes	2.700
Sousas	30.000
Joaquim Egidio	3.000
Good Hope	4.500
March 31st	5.000

According to the table above, it can be seen that the eastern region has around 250,000 inhabitants and, as mentioned, 70% depend exclusively on the SUS, which means that 175,000 people need health care and do not have any kind of private health care or health plan. According to the Oral Health Survey of 2010[59] (the last one carried out), the need for some kind of prosthesis starts at a very early age, from the age of 14, which leads us to think of the large number of people in this universe of 175,000 who depend on the prosthesis service.

In the municipality there have been prosthesis services since 2004, initially only for the elderly population (over 60), but without an evaluation of their functioning and efficiency. Is rehabilitating these users just restoring the physiological functions of the mouth? Wouldn't it be necessary to give them back their lost part(s), such as mutilation, suffering and exclusion? Give them their mouth back? This is also what we want to analyze in this research.

Pinheiro et al (2010, p.22)[87] point out that they have already identified countless experiences of implementing the SUS with innovative power, presenting different and progressive standards of integrality and equity, the result of democratic interactions of subjects in their practices of care management and social control:

(...) it is precisely in this innovative power that we find the constituent links of comprehensiveness practices, because in it lies a posture of active listening to demands, through voices whose ethical implication is the production of health as a right of citizenship.

In December 2004, the Municipality of Campinas' Oral Health Technical Area released its Management Report and, in its final remarks, highlights the fact that all the Health Teams (Reference Teams) have an oral health professional. But how does this professional provide care, listen, take anamneses and bond with the patient? And does he or she produce "experiences of implementing the SUS"? These are also questions that won't be answered in this work, but which must necessarily be present in our minds so that we can analyze the involvement of the professional who is also the researcher ....

In fact, special care was taken to carry out the interviews, as most of the users had already been seen by me. As I said in Chapter I, I have always enjoyed talking to patients, listening to their stories, and this creates a bond between us.

But Campos (2003, p.25)[6] states that there will be no possibility of establishing a bond between the team and the user if it is not clear how the team operates and, without a doubt, I have always operated in this way, trying to make the meetings "encounters".

In general, promotion and prevention is done "on" users and not "with" their active participation. Action on people and not with their involvement (...). As a result, programs lose their effectiveness when they try to manipulate and control people's desires, interests and values, according to the needs of norms established by epidemiology or political or administrative logic.

Cecilio (2001, p. 113)[88] points out that health needs present "a potentiality that would help workers, staff, services and service networks to listen better to the people who seek health care, taking the needs at the center of their interventions and practices", aiming for more humanized and qualified care.

In order to do this, it is necessary to welcome, promote a safe diagnosis and interfere in the evolution of suffering, re-establishing bodily homeostasis and producing a bond, the result of dialog, the assumption of responsibility and the resolution of the individual's complaints and needs (Barros and Botazzo, 2011)[33]. Simply restoring the teeth (through prostheses) of mutilated teeth is not enough to solve/improve users' quality of life...

When thinking about the production of health care, work management is a challenge. You have to understand the activities (situations), without excluding the possibility of a modification, or even a renunciation of a personal point of view. In other words, "health needs require a capacity for listening, respect for human, cultural and social diversity and an understanding of health and illness, as well as opportunities to build proposals for ways to change the clinic". (Pinheiro, Guizardi, Machado and Gomes, 2010, p.28)[87]

The institutionalization of the Dental Prosthesis Service and its impact on the users who benefit from it, have benefited from it or are waiting for it is the focus of this study. We want to investigate the viewpoint of those who have had their teeth mutilated throughout their lives and who therefore need prostheses. The assumptions include the oral problems most relevant to the users and how they were solved (or not). After all, there are more than three million elderly Brazilians who need full dentures in both arches and another four million who need partial dentures, according to SB Brasil 2010[59] and a large proportion of these users belong to the SUS in Campinas, which is the location of our study.

OBJECTIVES:

General

To analyze the process of institutionalization of a dental prosthesis service in the municipality of Campinas/SP, taking into account the municipality's health policy, the structuring of services and care practices in the face of oral health needs from the point of view of the subject-patient.

Specifics

A) To identify the oral health aspects of mutilated tooth users who have used, are using or are waiting to use the Prosthesis Service of the Eastern District of the municipality of Campinas.

B) To understand the work process of the Prosthesis Service within the context of a Basic Health Unit and its implications.

C) To analyze the potential of the institution "Prosthesis Service of SUS Campinas" for users with mutilated teeth, from the perspective of the subject-patient.

D) To point out possibilities for improving the service so that it is more resolute and effective.

METHODOLOGICAL PATH

This is qualitative research, which, according to Minayo (2014)[89], is applied to the study of the stories, relationships, representations, beliefs, perceptions and opinions of the subjects. Still according to this author, "qualitative approaches are suitable for investigating delimited and focused groups and segments, social histories from the perspective of the actors, relationships and for analyzing discourses and documents" (Minayo, 2014, p.57)[89], exactly as in the case of our research.

Pope and Mays (2005)[90] state that qualitative research is often defined by reference to quantitative research, as its methods are seen as the antithesis of quantitative or statistical methods, but they believe that, more than this, qualitative research does not simply accept numbers, concepts or explanations, but questions and investigates the nature of phenomena, especially social phenomena. They also state that instead of quantitative and qualitative approaches being seen as methodological opposites, each can be seen as complementary to the other.

These same authors conclude that, in general, the methods used in qualitative research include direct observation, interviews, analysis of texts or documents and of speeches or behaviors, but there is a common focus on speech and action, rather than on numbers.

Barros, Cecatti and Turato (2005)[91] believe that the multiplicity of perspectives, techniques, methods, knowledge and approaches of qualitative research are beneficial for understanding the phenomena linked to individuals in the health-disease process. It also allows us to better contextualize in order to think about, propose, test and recommend alternatives for health.

In fact, bringing the discourse about the "other" and not just the "numerical data" reaffirms the alterity that remains attentive to differences and singularities, helping to put the biomedical model and its interventions in parentheses.

According to Robert Stake (2011, p.68)[86] :

A qualitative researcher tries to report on a few situational experiences, usually not very many... selects the activities and contexts that offer the possibility of understanding an interesting part of how things work.

The theoretical-methodological approach we will use will be Institutional Analysis, with the use of diaries kept by the researcher and interviews with mutilated dental users of the SUS Campinas who use, have used or are still waiting to use the Prosthesis Service of the municipality.

L'Abbate (2012)[64], p.198 assumes that "Institutional Analysis aims to understand a given social and organizational reality, based on the discourses and practices of the subjects". To this end, it uses a method made up of an articulated set of concepts, including *order, demand, transversality, analyzer and implication.* When the analysis is carried out in situ, by a third party responding to an order, it is called *Socioanalysis.* When the material to be analysed is made up of documents, observations, interviews, it is called a *paper analysis* (as it will be in our case) and, for this, there is a professional (in this case, the researcher) who will be the expert in order to provide a diagnosis, in other words, an analysis of the demands that will elucidate problems in the organization. Thus, A.I. can be "didactically divided" into socio-analysis or socio-clinical; schizoanalysis and socio-psychoanalysis. And within socio-analysis, we have role analysis, socio-historical AI and intervention research.

In order to understand the theoretical and social genesis of what is known as Institutional Analysis (IA), the beginnings of which date back to the 1940s and 1950s, we must emphasize that:

The context of this production is, on the one hand, the broader political-ideological and scientific-intellectual crisis that French society was going through at the time, a crisis which also included the questioning of the internal workings of various organizations and the search for ways of acting to transform them. According to one of its main founders, René Lourau, it was about "transforming in order to know" and not the other way around, as is generally proposed by the most common approaches in the social sciences (L'Abbate, 2013. p.34).[7]

There is a consensus among scholars that A.I. had its theoretical foundation thanks to authors such as René Lourau, Georges Lapassade and Félix Guattari. L'Abbate (2012)[64] believes there are differences between them, as Lourau and Lapassade remained together in the field of A.I. and Socioanalysis and worked in universities, while Guattari was never linked to the academic world. In addition, their work differed theoretically and methodologically, even between Lourau and Lapassade. Each followed their own path.

Lourau (2004)[19] also stated that AI should be understood as deciphering what is hidden. He presents the *analyzer* as the one who reveals what is hidden and carries out the analysis in the institution, as mentioned above in Chapter IV.

Institutional Analysis (IA) and Collective Health (CH) have undergone transformations over time, but there is a coincidence between the two processes: an innovative/institutional character in relation to the existing body of knowledge and practices in their respective fields. (L'Abbate,2013)[7] .

When talking about the institutional nature of Collective Health in the 1960s, as discussed in the introduction to this paper, we need to "define" the word *"institutional"*. It comes from the concept of **Institution,** which according to Lourau (1975) and L'Abbate (1997, p.3)[92] is:

...visible social form endowed with legal and/or material organization, for example, a company, a school, a hospital, the industrial system, the school system, the hospital system of a country are called institutions. (...) It is more accurate to say that, dialectically analyzed, they break down into three moments": The **instituted** or the established, considered the moment of universality; the **instituting, that** is, the event that never ceases to alter and even negate what is formalized, which is particularity; and the third moment, that of singularity, the result of the articulation between the previous moments, which tends towards the daily practices of the subjects, producing something that is not merely reproductive and repetitive, but, on the contrary, points towards a certain actualization, a "becoming" in continuous transformation. This is the third moment, called **institutionalization.**

Thus, according to Lourau (2004)[19] , institutions are norms and include the way in which individuals agree, or not,

in participating in these same norms. This same author considered every institution "from wages to marriage" to be the result of the articulation between three moments: *The instituted* or moment of universality, as the institution is recognized and named; *the instituting* or moment of particularity that negates the previous moment; and *the institutionalization* or moment of singularity that is the result of the previous others, as transcribed in the quote above, when the institution is tensioned and actualized in the action of the subjects that constitute it.

Institutions have been defined as systems of rules that determine the lives of individuals, and can also refer to political constitutions, laws, fashions, superstitions, etc.

Two concepts from AI were used to understand the institutional context of this study: institution and implication. The concept of institution is what allows us to consider the Municipal Department's Oral Health Policy as an institution, with the prosthesis service being one of the ways in which this institution materializes, where its three dialectically related moments take place: the instituted or established, the instituting, or what is in motion, renewing the 1st moment and institutionalization as the result of the relationship between the previous moments.

The implication, which was already dealt with in Chapter I, concerns the fact that we are always relating, from an affective, ideological and professional point of view, to our object of study and to the institutions in which we are inserted. In the case of this research, the researcher's involvement was undoubtedly of great importance in choosing the Prosthesis Service where she works as the site of the investigation.

In order to analyze these implications, it was essential to draw up a research diary, a diary which, according to Lourau, is the researcher's narrative in its historical context, as it allows the researcher to reflect on their daily experiences.

The research diary provides an insight into the day-to-day experience of the field. The idea, then, was to use the diary as an instrument of observation/reporting/memories of what was being produced, or of what was happening throughout the research, an exercise in observing the behavior of a social group (in our case, a group of mutilated teeth).

Even more than describing experiences, the diary served as "an intervention tool". According to Pezzato and L'Abbate (2011, p.1303)[93] :

... the diary, from an AI perspective, is an intervention tool that has the

potential to produce a movement of reflection on one's own practice, insofar as the act of writing down what is experienced, whether individually or collectively, is the moment of reflection, revealing the unsaid and presupposing the non-neutrality of the researcher in the research process.

The narrative produced by the diary was combined with interviews with the mutilated teeth who had used, were using or were waiting to receive their prostheses from the Prosthesis Service. The aim of these interviews was to build up the users' *Pathografic Histories*, which we'll talk about later.

According to Pezzato and L'Abbate (2011)[93] , if we set out to write a research diary, we will be exercising written language, exposing our professional-social-cultural-indigenous weaknesses, in other words, analyzing the dimensions of our involvement. Reflecting on our own "action-intervention" in our daily work.

So, to keep a diary is to stop and reflect, to analyze the moment, to dive into the implications and try, in some way, to generate a movement.

Mendes, Pezzato and Sacardo (2016)[94] , state that when we write a diary, we become subjects of the writing process and this requires a willingness to review, to let ourselves be touched by the experience and to reflect on it. According to these authors, the diary is a document of what was experienced, it is a record of what was possible to report at the time and, therefore, with contradictions, doubts, conflicts and joys.

Finally, Pezzato and L'Abbate (2011, p. 1311)[93] conclude that the methodological use of diaries makes it possible to see other ways of intervening, insofar as "... when the diarist wrote or reported on what they experienced, they had to elaborate on how a particular action took place, taking it out of the natural scene of everyday life and putting it up for discussion and reflection."

In our case, the diary was also an instrument for analyzing our involvement throughout the research process. Often, we even noticed over-implication, which forced us to stop and (re)stop, change course...

The line of research that "analyzes institutions" (A.I.), developed in France in the 1960s and 1970s, formulated the idea of "intervention research" which, according to Passos and Benevides de Barros (2000)[95] aims to interrogate the meanings crystallized in institutions.

Passos and Barros (2000)[95] also understand that, in the context where clinic and politics intersect, the word intervention joins research not to replace action, but to produce another way of relating theory and practice, as well as subject and object.

Barbier (2002)[96], working with action research, refers to a "spiral approach that implies a recursive effect as a result of permanent reflection on action".

More recently, Pezzato and L'Abbate (2012 p.132)[97] brought a strategy that addresses the relationship between action research and intervention research:

What we propose is to stimulate a dialogue by explaining the uniqueness of the combination of the two approaches (action research and intervention research) ... The aim is to articulate research, reflection, action, theory, practice, intervention, clinical practice, politics, subjects, desires..., demonstrating a strong interrelationship between the two.

The style of research known as action research is particularly suitable for identifying problems in clinical practice and helping to develop potential solutions in order to improve practice, according to Pope and Mays (2005)[90] and this is our idea.

It is more a style of research than a specific method. It was first used by Kurt Lewin in 1946, a social scientist concerned with relations and minorities in the USA. Childs (1997)[98] states that "Action research is now identified as research in which researchers work explicitly *with* and *for* people rather than conducting research *on* them (emphasis added).

Finally, Rocha and Aguiar (2003)[99] include action research and intervention research as participatory research and conclude that in both, the subjects are involved and it is therefore impossible to maintain neutrality.

Again quoting Pezzato and L'Abbate (2012, p.136)[97] "the form of the research, whether action research or intervention research, will depend on the strong interaction between the participants in the work" and this is how we hoped to conduct this research.

The authors also consider that both are ways of approaching the micropolitics of everyday life in health services and that "the debate around the need to demarcate, or not, the spaces/territories of each of them is open."

In addition to the diaries, a useful tool of the IA, we conducted interviews with users who had used or were using the service and also with some of those on the "waiting lists".

For Haguette (2013, p. 81)[100] the interview can be defined as:

A process of interaction between two people in which one of them, the interviewer, aims to obtain information from the other, the interviewee. The information is obtained through an interview script consisting of a list of points or topics previously established according to a central problem and which must be followed.

In our work, the aim of these interviews was to construct/elaborate pathografic histories of users so that analysis could be carried out.

Historia Patogrâfica is a fusion of Castiel's concept of clinical history[101] - which combines the factual and fictional dimensions of clinical history - and Lain Entralgo's concept of pathography[102] - which proposes describing the patient and their life beyond the clinical aspects (Kovaleski and Freitas, 2010)[103] . It is a powerful tool that suggests a deeper understanding of the lived experience, as in our case.

Castiel (1994)[101] merges fictional accounts (stories and accounts of events) with stories and proposes the theoretical formulation of clinical stories, which are narratives produced by patients, who seek coherence between their ideas of themselves and their surroundings, seeking compatibility with the medical histories collected. In short, it's about interpreting content and constructing meanings.

Entralgo (1998)[102] brings a significant contribution from psychoanalysis to the clinic. He places the concern with ordering the illness in the patient's biography and, in this way, the pathographic report gains nuances that include the different ways in which the patient conceives of the illness. This author opposes the clinical history, which is intended as a neutral account. In this way, it has a different perspective on the clinic and, thus, the "cold" clinical report of a health condition gives way to the illness perceived in a subjective and singular way.

To this end, this study intends to pay special attention to the interviews and the transcriptions, taking care to make each interviewee's story come alive. Their feelings and perceptions surrounding tooth loss and the effects on their lives.

We used the methodology of pathographic stories, an instrument proposed by Souza (2003)[44] , which presents the technique of reporting field research, especially dedicated to interviews, where the transcript is partially used, giving way to the researcher's live report, interspersed with the statements of the individuals interviewed.

The instruments of clinical practice wisdom will be used to organize the narratives, with interpretative questions being asked by the researcher.

After approval by the FCM/Unicamp Research Ethics Committee (Opinion No. 1.668.950), 18 patients were selected, six of whom were on the waiting list with inadequate prostheses that needed replacing, or without any prostheses at all; six users who had already completed their prostheses at the aforementioned service and six who were in the process of being seen/consulted for prostheses.

All 18 interviewees (except for one who died) agreed to collaborate/participate in the study, were informed about the objectives, signed the informed consent form (ICF) and kept a copy of it. They were also able to choose the date, time and place of the interviews (their homes or the Health Center).

As far as possible, the selection process respected the proportionality of sex and age of the total number of patients.

The interviews were recorded and then faithfully transcribed. They were then analyzed in parallel with the entries in the diaries, with close dates or old diaries, but with similar themes/subjects, in order to observe distances, conjugations and approximations, according to the "essay" by Pezzato and Prado (2013)[104] .

The semi-structured, open-ended interviews included questions aimed at retracing the interviewees' lives prior to their tooth loss. To this end, the interviewees were asked about their experiences with oral health care during three phases of their lives: childhood, adolescence and adulthood.

Each phase was defined chronologically by the interviewee. The interviewees' narratives related to oral health care were sought. How they took care of it, who took care of it, if there was any

outstanding memory. At each moment, they were asked about their contact with the health service(s) and their perception of it.

People were made as comfortable as possible so that they could freely narrate their experiences. They were only interrupted when they needed to explain something in relation to a gesture, expression...

In this way, we hoped to get to know the situation in which the mutilated tooth users found themselves and involve them in the process. During the interviews we problematized so that the participants would perceive the need for change (or not) and would want to play an active role both in the research and in the process of transformation (or not).

The Prosthetic Service of the Eastern District

We made a cut and stipulated a period from October 2007 to October 2015 so that we could count the various prostheses made, for various patients, of different ages and sexes, from the 10 different regions (UBSs) that refer users to this prosthesis service, as shown in the table below.

The ages were stratified into age groups as suggested by the World Health Organization (WHO) for sample composition, namely: 15 to 19 years; 35 to 44 years and 65 to 74 years. This same pattern is used by the Projeto Saùde Bucai (SB) Brasil 2010[59] which is the most up-to-date report on the oral health conditions of the Brazilian population.

Table 02: Ratio of the age group and sex of the patients who underwent used prostheses from October 2007 to October 2015.

Age range		Female	Male	Total (age group)
Young	15 to 19 years old	48	39	87
Adult	35 to 44 years old	205	111	316
Elderly	65 to 74 years old	245	180	425
Over 74	> 74 years	98	53	151
	Total (by gender)	596	383	979

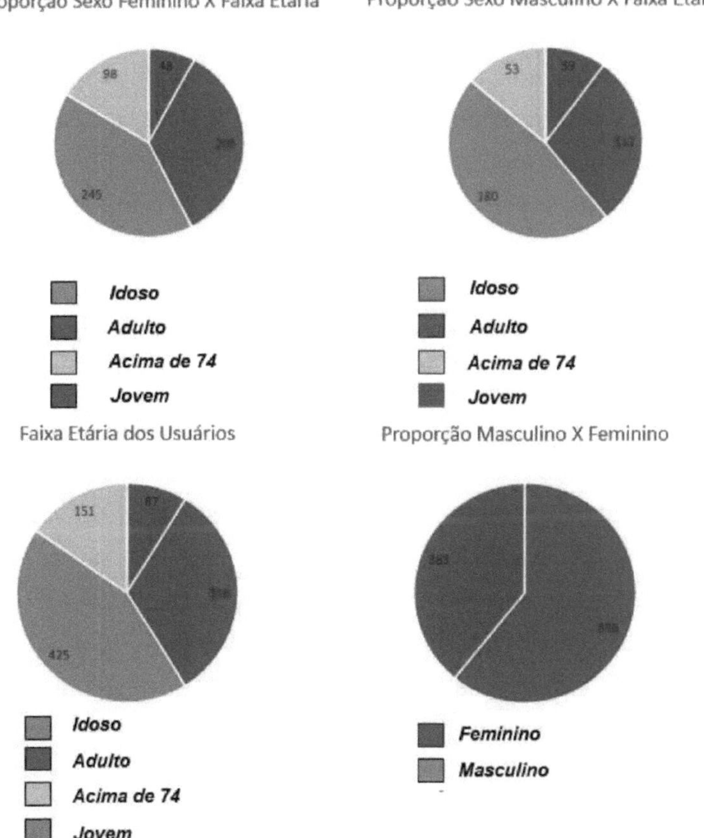

It can be seen that women are in the majority and that the age group that was most often in the service during the period studied was the "elderly phase", i.e. male and female patients between 65 and 74 years old. There is a bias in this data, because when we took over the service we only carried out prostheses for the elderly. Our perception today is that there is an equivalence between the "adult phase and the elderly phase".

A recent article published in the journal of the Paulista Association of Dental Surgeons (APCD Journal - February 2016)[105] states that tooth loss is progressive and has been getting earlier and earlier. He adds that 28% of young adults have no functional teeth in at least one of their arches. In the light of this data, it is clear that this group of the population needs some kind of prosthesis, which confirms our perception of the day-to-day demand for the service.

Over the ten years I've been in charge of the service, I've noticed that there are an average of 350 users on the "waiting list" at the Costa e Silva Health Center alone (one of the ten UBS that refer prostheses). If we consider that 2 to 3 patients are called every 2 months, we realize that we start with around 20 to 30 patients per call period, but it takes an average of 2 to 3 months to complete the work. Thus, on average, we see 12 patients a month, which is very little compared to the demand/need.

Specifically in the Eastern District, we work without any help, in other words, there is no oral health technician (TSB) or oral health assistant (ASB). These professionals could speed up the service by making phone calls to schedule or reschedule appointments (when for some reason there is no service due to lack of material, or equipment breakdown, or loss of service during transportation, or exchange in the laboratory itself, duplicate scheduling, among others). Filling in forms, making return appointments, pouring plaster, handling the impression material (plaster or zinc enolic paste), organizing the bench, cleaning the equipment between patients, packing the prostheses so that they arrive properly at the laboratory, checking the boxes that are returned after the laboratory services have been carried out, in short, tasks that are the responsibility of these professionals and that would certainly optimize the dentist's time, and could then expand access by opening up more hours to be made available for new patients in need of prostheses.

In addition to the absence of the TSB and ASB, there is no replacement for the professional when she is on vacation or premium leave. As a result, for a period of two months a year, no prostheses are made or those that have already been made.

Another point to be mentioned is the return visits for adjustments after the services have been delivered, because it is often only after daily use that places that rub against the mucosa are noticed and can form lesions. These two or three returns could be made at the primary care unit, by the dentist who made the referral to the prosthesis service, which would optimize the schedule even more, making room for other new patients in need of rehabilitation.

Finally, we would like to point out that the location of the prosthesis laboratory is not in the municipality itself. The managers opted not to have a laboratory (as suggested by the National Oral Health Policy) and a bidding process was opened via "electronic tender" for outsourcing. In the 10 years that we have been in the service, we have already had laboratories accredited in the municipalities of Jaguariuna (SP), Curitiba (PA), Sâo Pulo (Capital) and currently in Campo Bello (MG).

Below I transcribe one of the documents that was drawn up and sent to the Municipality's Oral Health Coordination, so that they could be informed, with the aim of clarifying the reality experienced and all the problems and inconveniences that occurred due to the distance/location of the prosthesis laboratory.

Campinas, February 14, 2013

Costa e Silva Health Center

East District Prosthesis Service Reference Headquarters

In a recent meeting with the coordinator of this Basic Health Unit, we thought it would be good to share some of the situations that have been occurring since the beginning of the Municipal Health Department's current contract with the

Prosthesis Laboratory of Curitiba, which was accredited after a bidding process.

Although we have been communicating informally (by phone and e-mail), we want to document the unforeseen events that have hindered the smooth running of this service:

1) Deadlines not met by the laboratory, leading to multiple rescheduling of patients' appointments. Often we are unable to communicate with the necessary advance notice, which creates considerable discomfort, as well as transportation costs for those who come and are not seen due to the service not arriving by post.

2) Errors in sending work, resulting in services being received from patients who don't belong to this District and the loss of our services, which sometimes go to other Districts.

3) Error in the packaging of services, resulting in a box with a name label that does not coincide with the bearer of the service included in the box.

4) Making "bases" (the prosthesis test stage) out of unsuitable and outdated material (Shillingburg, Hobo and Whitsett, 1990), leading to fractures and wasted time and materials to repeat the stage in question.

5) Breakages/fractures and dismantling during transportation, since the laboratory in question is in Curitiba (Paranà) and the "suitcases" are sent by post and/or "motorcycle boy" when they go to Suzano.

6) Return of services without execution of the work requested from the

This frustrates the patient, who often waits around 15 days to try on their prosthesis, but the prosthesis returns at the same stage as it was sent...

We understand that this is an evaluative moment, necessary as a diagnostic tool about the organization (structure) and functioning (process), with the aim (results) of improving things for everyone involved.

We thank you and remain at your disposal for any further clarification you may require.

The document was signed by me and the local coordinator of the Unit and filed with the town hall. We received no response. A very significant **analysis of** the importance given to the service by managers...

After many reports, phone calls, other emails, and documents, such as the one transcribed above, a meeting was scheduled (on July 22, 2013, at the Campinas Dental Surgeons Association - ACDC - note that the document above was dated February 14) with the representatives of the laboratory, the 5 supporters of the respective districts, the 5 dental surgeons who make the prostheses and the municipality's Oral Health coordinator.

On this occasion, everyone had the opportunity to speak and, after many regrets, the coordinator himself made a statement to the effect that it was not possible to continue with the contract in this way. So some agreements were made and a three-month deadline set for a re-evaluation.

In fact, some steps were taken, including the hiring of a laboratory right here in Campinas to carry out some of the phases and another laboratory in Suzano for other laboratory phases, as already mentioned. It's worth noting that these were "drawer" contracts, as they were signed not by the municipality, but by the Curitiba laboratory itself, as a way of solving the huge problems reported at the meeting (including the delay in delivery deadlines).

Some unforeseen events, such as an accident involving the "motoboy" who was picking up and bringing back the boxes containing the prostheses, on the Suzano-Campinas route, and robberies of the post office cars that were taking the packages to Curitiba, with the consequent disappearance of the prostheses, were new inherent events that had serious consequences for us, but in fact the technical quality of the services improved.

The re-evaluation meeting, which should have taken place after three months, never took place ...

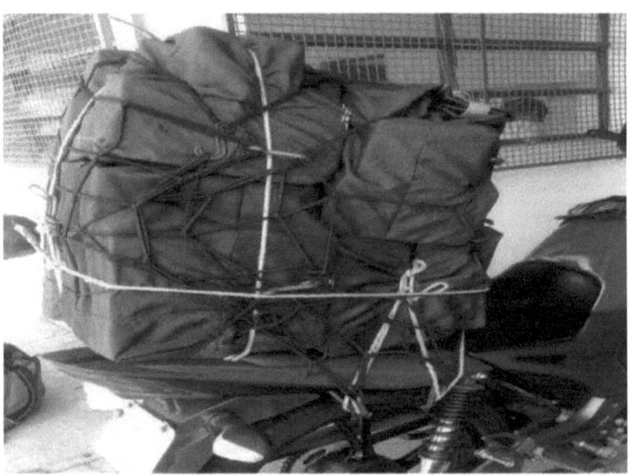

Image 1- An overcrowded motorcycle with almost no room for the driver. This was the precarious way in which the suitcases containing the prostheses were transported from the city of Campinas to Suzano (S.P.), after the outsourced laboratory had hired another location to carry out some of the stages.

Patients who had their prosthetic pieces missing/stolen had to restart the first impression process, generating frustration, overloading the schedule (new patients were not called), not to mention the extra expense, since the municipality had to pay for the restart of the new prostheses that had to be made again.

CHAPTER VI: SOME PATHOLOGICAL STORIES:

Of the 979 prostheses completed in the period in question (between 2007 and 2015), we selected 18 users for interviews and the subsequent preparation of pathogrpahy histories. We tried, as far as possible, to maintain equivalence between male and female patients and age groups, as shown in the table below.

Table 3: Users in the process of having prostheses made, users with prostheses already completed and users on the waiting list

	Name	Sex	Age range
Users in process clothing prostheses	Nice Guy	Male	>74 years (82 years)
	Mr. Crutches	Male	>74 years (78 years)
	Ombudsman	Male	Elderly (71 years old)
	Mrs. Poli complaining	Female	Elderly woman (68 years old)
	Community Agent	Female	Adult (36 years old)
	Boy from the Chàcara	Female	Young (30 years old)
Users with their own theses already completed	Mr. swollen feet	Male	>74 years (83 years)
	Mrs. Warrior	Female	Elderly woman (63 years old)
	Young Believer	Male	Adult (52 years old)
	Cancer boy	Male	Adult (56 years)
	Mrs. Banguela	Female	Young (25 years old)
	Cashier	Female	Young (22 years old)
Users on the waiting	Stroke Lady	Female	>74 years (78 years)
	Ponte Preta fan	Female	>74 years (78 years)
	Mr. Died	Male	Elderly (68 years old)
	Mr. Talking	Male	Elderly (65 years)
	Mr. Boiling	Male	Adult (49 years old)
	Mr. "Not long now	Male	Adult (45 years)

1. "Nice Guy"

Mr. G.S.A. is 82 years old and very healthy. He is the grandson of Mrs. "M", who was treated here at the Health Center until she was placed in a home for the elderly, due to Alzheimer's and Mr. G. no longer being able to take care of her alone. He knows everyone, talks to everyone in the corridors, waits to be called into the consulting rooms, always "striking up" a conversation with the other patients who are also waiting to be called. He had been on the waiting list for several years because he wanted to replace his upper denture. The father of three children and grandfather to five grandchildren, he tells us about his life with great joy. When I invited him to do the interview, he was so happy. It was like an invitation to a wedding...

He was born right here in the city and was a "little guard" at the Dako stove factory. Tell us about it:

"It's not your time... You weren't even born... now the factory is bankrupt. The big brands have swallowed it up... but that's where I started my professional life. I learned the trades and worked my way up to head of department, where I retired. The salary wasn't great

thing, but I raised the three children and I have my own little house. The "M" Clinic [referring to the clinic where his wife is hospitalized] is very expensive, something for a "big shot", which is why my children help me pay for it. We wanted to put her in a very good place. The children went to a government school, but it was very good. Now it's all rubbish.... Then everyone went to work and had their own lives, but there was never a shortage of food at home. We only gave them toys at Christmas, but why else? They played in the street, played ball, ihhhh... life was good! M" [referring to the eldest son] was the only one who went to university, because at PUC those who work during the day can study at night for free. So he graduated, right? Now he's earning a good salary, but he's fallen in love with another woman, and now he's in trouble because the other woman wants a pension. And he has to give it, right? It's the right thing to do. The children are with her, she has to buy food, pay for clothes and shoes...

Now his salary will be cut short because he'll have to support them both. I just want to see.... The smartest one, he even has a diploma, but he's on a roll..."

When I asked him about the difficulty of losing his teeth, he answered very naturally:

"-My daughter, I'm 82 years old. I've lost my teeth throughout my life and I've had to get used to it, like everything else you lose... because I never had the money to go to a private dentist and at the clinic they just pulled them out, as I've already told you. They never came up with anything. I was very poor and at that time there were no cheap dentists. So a dentist was only for rich people.... You either had to get your teeth done at the post office, or go to a city that did fillings. When you had to put in a "pivot" it was expensive, so we had it pulled out. We took good care of our teeth. In our own way, because we didn't have the things we have today: toothbrushes of all sizes, good toothpaste, mouthwash... ih- hhh, today there's everything, not in our time. And so it went on, one tooth, another, until I had none. Then I got these dentures, but I'm quite old now, I must be about 20 years old, so I put my name on the list and waited to find a place... Now, I'm going to wait a bit longer until the dentures arrive, because there's no way around it, right? You have to make the molds, you have to send them to Curitiba [the city that had an agreement with the prosthetics laboratory accredited by the Campinas municipal government, the site of the research]. I understand, you've already explained all this to me... I've waited a long time in this life. Do what, right????" [referring to the delay in getting the new prosthesis ready, as it was in the process of being made].

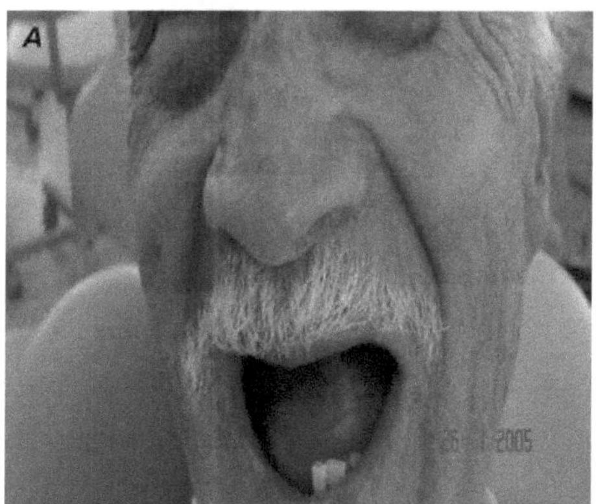

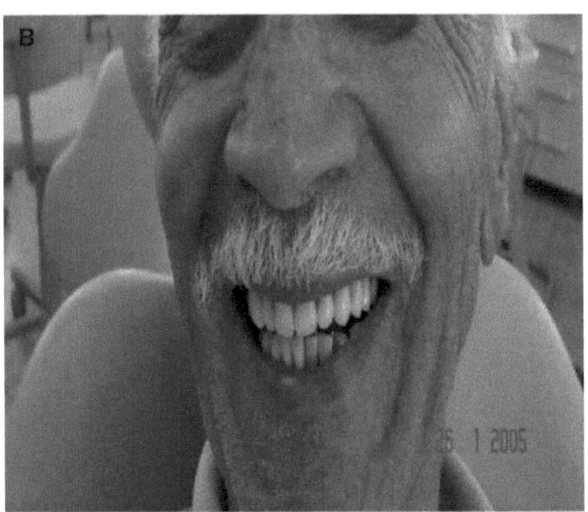

Image 2 A and B: "Simpàtico Senhorzinho before (A) - with only 3 elements in his mouth: teeth from inequality and the marks of a poor and difficult life, and after (B) the making of a new upper total prosthesis and a lower partial prosthesis.

2. "Lord of Crutches"

Patient was born on 21/01/1939, in Espirito Santo do Pinhal and came to Campinas as a child with his parents and younger brother, "A". This brother is now his carer, because Mr. de Muletas suffered a stroke and is left with several sequelae: he practically can't move the left side of his body; he walks with difficulty, using crutches; he also speaks with difficulty and spends almost all his time lying down, because that's how he feels best. Sitting up gives him a lot of pain. He tells me that he had six siblings, but only the two who were still small came with their parents to Campinas. They wanted to try for a better life.... He currently takes Captopril and Alodipine continuously. Despite so many difficulties, he lives alone because he separated from his wife more than 30 years ago and has only one daughter, who is married. He has two granddaughters and lives in Hortolândia. When it comes to eating, he chooses more pasty foods, such as bananas, papaya, soft bread, yoghurt, noodles, "miojo", among others, because he only has two teeth left in his mouth and he also has a lot of difficulty/limitations when it comes to cooking.

I asked him about his childhood in Espirito Santo de Pinhal and, perhaps because he knew about my profession, he began to talk about his oral health and said that when he was a child his teeth were good: "I didn't have any bad ones and I cleaned them myself with a brush and paste. When I needed a dentist for any reason, there was one in Pinhal who did the job and marked it in his notebook. But I had to take a lot of antibiotics after I came to Campinas because I had "Asian fever" and this ruined my teeth. We had a lot of difficulties here, because the locals had their noses to the grindstone and didn't mix with outsiders. So it wasn't easy to get a job and even the Culto à Ciência College only accepted pupils if they were the children of rich people," she said with sadness in her eyes.

He also told me that he lost his teeth because "pus bubbles" began to form on his gums and he had to have them extracted. There were no health centers, only one, in Orozimbo Maia, and there was no dentist, so it was necessary to borrow money to be able to "pull them out". He said: "A private dentist was very expensive and they looked down on us and then said they didn't have the time. The way was to look for more popular clinics. If it was fifty reais at the private clinic, we'd get it for ten. When we felt a lot of pain, the health center would give us an injection that we couldn't feel for three days." Since then, she has only two remaining teeth in her lower arch.

His brother is the one who has been telling him this whole story and Mr. de Muletas has been nodding in agreement the whole time, but he is starting to feel unwell, he is sweating and complains of being too stuffy/hot and suspects that his blood pressure is rising.... At this point, we interrupted the interview and asked a nursing assistant to take his blood pressure: 170 x 112mm Hg. The brother asks Mr. de Muletas if he has taken his medication and he replies that "the right time to take it is only at 10:00".

I recline my chair a little to try to make him more comfortable and wait a while, but I decide to finish the interview on another day so that he can return home, take his medication and rest.

We agreed to finish at another time.

Today "Lord on crutches" returned with his brother for the installation of the prostheses. A full upper prosthesis and a partial lower prosthesis ("bridge"). It took 9 sessions of coming and going to test and repair the distortions and problems. The model also had to be re-molded because it was broken on the way from Campinas to Curitiba (the location of the laboratory contracted by the municipality). He was then very anxious, reporting that he had already prepared several times to go home with his "new teeth". He told me that he had made a soup, as instructed by us, because he wants to adapt quickly to the prostheses. I explain that we're going to try it out, test the occlusion and the adaptation and then I'll give him a mirror... He smiles and says he likes surprises, but doesn't hide his tension. I make the clinical adjustments and give him a mirror, which he holds up with difficulty. When he sees himself, his eyes fill with tears; he apologizes, says it's the emotion. "I've lost everything in my life, my wife, my daughter and my granddaughters, who are very far away from me..." He also lost the possibility of autonomy, the movement of his legs and arms, his teeth... and now at least he's got his teeth back... he's happy!

I explain to him that speech and chewing will be difficult at first and that it will be necessary to remove the prostheses to carry out hygiene after every meal, which will be an additional task in his life, but one that is totally necessary to prevent the accumulation of residues and micro-organisms (which can be deposited on the palate due to the hot and humid environment). It will also be necessary to knead the food, which should be thickened slowly as you feel more confident and secure, and finally, I am at your disposal for adjustments and wear on the prostheses, should they hurt.

She got up with great difficulty, with the help of me and her brother, leaning on her crutches and thanking us. He leaves and says goodbye to everyone in the room:

God bless you for the beautiful work you do!

The "Lord of Crutches" came back the next day and we talked some more. He told me that it was really good when he had his teeth, but these (referring to the prostheses) were even nicer and that he had already realized that they were very "sharp" and that he could therefore go back to eating healthier food... "I couldn't take soup and bread any more... Now I can eat meat! ".

We talked about the process of making the prostheses and he seemed to have forgotten all the inconveniences he had been through. The five protocol sessions turned into nine (almost twice as long as planned)[13] and, as a result, he ended up waiting almost six months to finally receive them, but his satisfaction with his new smile left no room for bad memories.

Daily of 22/10/2011

"I'm glad I'm going on vacation. Lately I've been feeling a bit depressed.

When the time comes to leave the house to go to the C.S., I'm already feeling desperate... I wonder what the problem is today. One day there's a shortage of plaster, the next day there's no molding paste, the next day the schedule has two patients at the same time and I end up having to see both of them because I can't just take one and send it away.... It's not their fault.... Not to mention the prosthesis laboratory, which we're tired of complaining about and asking to change, but it's still in Curitiba... Where have you seen that? All this distance and technical and organizational incompetence. They don't meet deadlines and we have to reschedule patients. They send the boxes with the names changed (I go to try on Mr. José's prosthesis and it doesn't fit because it's not actually his, and I don't know whose it is...), not to mention the losses (the pieces "disappear" or go to another C.S.) and I end up restarting the work from the first impression."

---

13 *The researcher's diaries have been kept since Pezzato's doctoral research in 2009, through the period in which she took part in the research "Innovation in the Production of Oral Health Care: possibilities for a new approach in the dental clinic for the Unified Health System - mentioned in Chapter I - and throughout the course of this doctorate. Some fragments/excerpts from these diaries have been included here in order to note the recurrence of the same problems over all these years.*

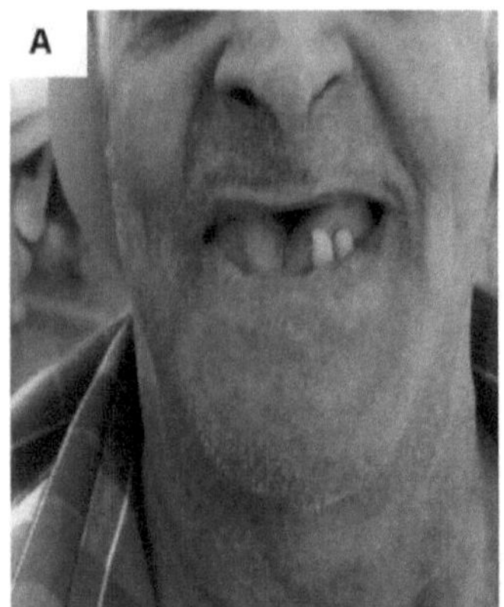
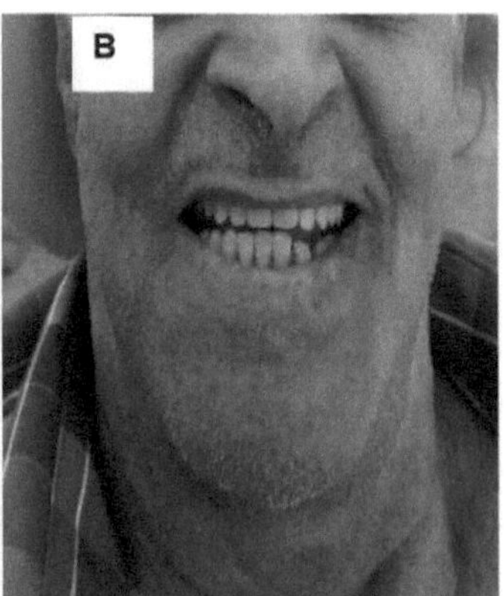

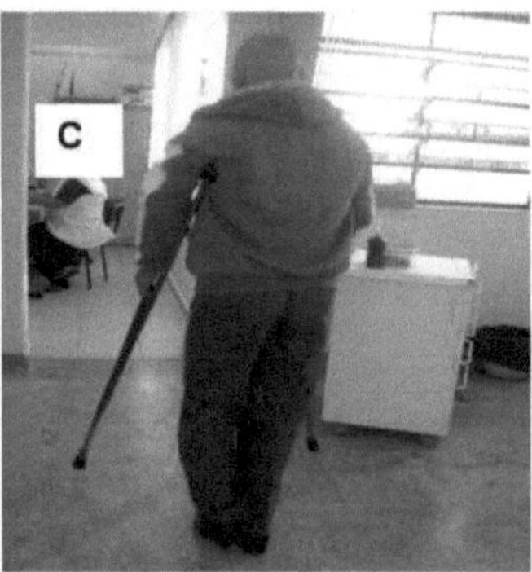

Image 3 A and B: Man on crutches before (A) - only two lower limbs: marks of difficulties and exclusion, and after (B) rehabilitation with total upper and partial lower prostheses. (C) Man on crutches leaving the room.

3. *"Ombudsman's man"*

I received a referral from the psychiatrist right here at the Health Center. Dr. "I" [the psychiatrist] asked for rehabilitation to improve the patient's self-esteem.

Mr. O.M., born on 14/06/46 here in Campinas. His mother was a manicurist and his father was a Bosch electrician. He never married and in his medical records we found notes from the psychologist who accompanied him during his adolescence. The report of shyness and introspection is frequent in the various consultations. He lives alone in a good house, although the community workers and the nurse have observed that there is a lot of dirt and an accumulation of broken and old objects.

We soon realized that he has upper and lower teeth in good condition. We also found reports in the file from the Unit's clinical dentist (various restorations, cleanings and some extractions). He speaks very little, hands us the referral and asks where he can sit [we have four dental chairs in the room]. I fill in the form with his personal details and try to start a friendly conversation to understand his medical history. He starts by saying that he wants to have his missing tooth fitted. He says that his mother has always brought him to the Health Center and that he's been to every dentist and doctor in the unit, each time a different one, and that they've all been good, but he had to have that tooth removed [he points to the edentulous space in the upper arch] because it broke and "couldn't be fixed".

I take the impressions and schedule a return appointment. The service didn't come back from the lab on the scheduled date, so we called to reschedule it. To our surprise, a few days later, we received a folder from the municipal ombudsman's office with a complaint from Mr. O.M. and we had to respond as soon as possible. (Case number 2315/2012. Subject 2380) It wasn't difficult to explain to the ombudsman that the prosthetics laboratory was outsourced and that we had no way of guaranteeing the deadlines, although there was a "protocol" of days expected for the services to be returned. At our second meeting, we talked about what had happened and Mr. O.M. told us that he had learned from his mother that by complaining to the ombudsman's office "things move faster... that's the way it is in the public service, it only works if we speak up".

We patiently explain how the service works and the difficulties we encounter along the way. I tell him that we're going to be together in the "fight" for rehabilitation and that, like him, we also want to see his smile "whole", without any missing teeth. He calms down and from then on the work went well.

He agreed to take part in the interview, saying:

"_ we have to do everything to get what is rightfully ours. I'll help you!"

He told us that he had always taken very good care of his teeth. His mother always took him to the health center and after her death she continued to take care of him. "The dentists would clean and fill his teeth, but sometimes his teeth would have a big cavity and he'd have to have a root canal, and after the root canal, sometimes he'd break his teeth eating something really soft, not even peanuts or hard meat. The ones at the back aren't missed, but this one at the front I don't want to be without. It broke at the root and Dr. "D" [referring to the Unit's dentist] took it out. Now I'm going to put in this bridge that you're going to make to put it back. There's no way I'm going to be without it."

I didn't want to take pictures.

4. "Mrs. Poli complaining"

Daily of 08/04/2014

One Monday morning, the local coordinator asked me to come to her office for a chat. I shuddered at the thought... what was it going to be???? It wasn't a scolding or a complaint, but a headache that's been with me for so long that I don't even know.... I can't stand to deal with S.T. anymore. Everything seems to go wrong with her. It seems that the more complicated the person, the more the service gets in trouble and doesn't move. It's been like this with her for the last three months. Everything that's already difficult gets worseWell,   R. (UBS coordinator) told me that

day that it wasn't going to be easy, but even so, she needed me to fit this patient in so that she'd be at ease. Well, she's given me peace of mind in coordination and a headache here in prosthetics. There isn't a single day when she comes in and the test goes well. There are always adjustments. Today was worse. I went to try it on and it wasn't her prosthesis. It was in her box, with her name on it, but it wasn't hers... Again there was

change in the lab... what now??? Where's the courage to say that I'm going to start all over again... or say that they've changed it and I know they'll never find it again... then, of course, she'll charge me and I'll go crazy... as if I were responsible for finding the lost/exchanged prosthesis. Did you go to another CS? To another city? I ended up telling the truth. There was an exchange of boxes and we don't know with which other box/other prosthesis/other person it was exchanged, so we don't know how we're going to destroy it or if we're going to find it. We're going to call Curitiba [the municipality that won the tender to carry out the laboratory phase of the prostheses] and see if they can find out... if they can't, we'll have to start all over again. She said she was going to complain to the District, that she was going to call the ombudsman, 156, talk to the coordinator... in the end, I thought it was good. Maybe now, if she really makes a fuss, they (the managers) will take action. Meanwhile, I'm stuck with my headache: I can't finish the prostheses and I can't get rid of her (patient). And even when I've finished, I'm sure she'll continue to bother me... She'll never be happy... God forbid, what a headache!

Born on April 1, 1949, she has lived in the neighborhood since she was born. They say her family was already very complicated. Her father drank a lot and never had a steady job. The mother made cakes and snacks for the outside, but didn't earn enough to keep the house, her daughter and younger brother. As a result, they had a lot of difficulties and on several occasions she had to be "rescued" by the staff of the Health Centre, who would mobilize and bring supplies and cleaning and hygiene materials. After her parents died, her unmarried brothers kept the house, but without any stability. They had only completed high school and, without specific training, it was difficult to earn more than the minimum wage.

When she started treatment with me, she worked as a clerk in the building materials store that was right outside the basement of the health center. She went out several times a day to try to get urgent care at the health center. According to the coordinator and the nursing assistants, her complaints were diverse. And indeed, during the rehabilitation treatment, this was confirmed. When I called her in the waiting room, I could already see her "closed face". One day her back hurt, the next her head, the next it was a "spur" in her foot or arthritis in her knees, and it was no different with her teeth. He told me in the interview that he always had problems with his teeth because they were "weak". She had them restored but still had pain. I treated the root canal and it still hurt, until I opted for extraction. But even for the extractions, she said she suffered a lot.

"The anesthesia didn't take, I bled a lot after I went home, the stitches came out before the right time, it got infected..." Anyway, it wasn't an easy case. The whole process took five months. Between comings and goings, appointments scheduled and sometimes canceled and sometimes rescheduled, we had to exercise calm and patience to deal with the various complaints and the endless complaints. She was invited to take part in the research and said she accepted because she wanted to collaborate with the service. She could see that I was involved and that's why she wasn't going to refuse. But the interview was too tiring. He spoke for almost two hours non-stop and never answered the questions directly. She complained the whole time about the pharmacy, which never had the medicine she was taking, the doctor who didn't even measure her blood pressure, the nurse who didn't feel like asking for a test and, of course, the dentists who didn't work, took too long to make an appointment and that she only got an appointment to have her prosthesis made because she went straight to the coordinator... Finally, she disappeared and we only heard from the nursing assistants. They told us that she didn't use the prostheses and that she said that "city hall services are always rubbish...

Patient didn't want to take photos...

5. *"Community Agent"*

V.C.C. has been our community health worker for over 18 years. She was born on 08/05/1981 in Limeira and came to Campinas as a child. Her father worked in the plantation, but she wanted to try for a better job here in the city. She studied until high school and helped her mother with sewing, until she was offered a job as a community health worker. She applied and was classified to work at the Costa e Silva Health Center. After passing the exam, she ended up marrying and has three children. She immediately accepted our invitation to take part in the research and made a point of welcoming us into her home one Saturday morning with delicious juice and cheese rolls.

I ask her to try not to confuse my position as a researcher with that of the CS dentist who is making her prosthesis, even though I know how difficult this can be.

I ask you to tell me about your childhood, your adolescence, your coming to Campinas and how you looked after your mouth.

He tells me that they were very poor and lived in a two-room house in the countryside of Limeira, on a farm where his father worked. There were five brothers and only their father worked as a farmer. His mother stayed at home to look after the children and the house. She cooked on a wood-burning stove everything they grew on the farm and made a lot of jam with the pumpkin and banana they had in large quantities in the yard. They also sucked sugar cane and believe that all these sweets were bad for their teeth. "We didn't brush, I think... I don't know, I don't remember. I don't think there was a toothbrush for everyone. There were one or two in the tank outside and sometimes we brushed..., but most days I don't think so..." They studied at the school group nearby and their father would take them there early in the morning in a buggy, but then they would walk back.

"When I was about 12, we came to Campinas and my father went to work at Pirelli. He managed to buy a house from "Coabi" and we felt like we were in paradise, because there was a room just for us [referring to the brothers] and a bathroom with a toilet and sink."

She met her husband at school and they dated for two years. Then she became pregnant with her first child and the father agreed to build a "little house" in the back so that they could live there.

Several times we are interrupted by children asking to sit on the sofa to play video games. She talks to her children, explaining that we are doing very important work. She says that if they continue to "grind", she'll take them to the clinic and have an injection given to each one... He tells them to go outside and play. After two or three requests, I suggest we go into the kitchen and I end up being applauded by the children.

"What a nice dentist..."

He tells his story and looks for reasons to explain the state of his mutilated mouth:

"- First there were the sweets from the farm. As I told you, we didn't even have a toothbrush. We didn't care about that. I sucked sugar cane, ate sweets that my mother made, I didn't care... It was only after we came to Campinas that I began to understand that I had to take care of it. At school, everyone thought it was ugly that we had bad teeth. Also, everything was black, right? So we went to the health center and fixed what we could. It's very well known, isn't it? Things aren't easy there.... Now that I work there it's difficult, imagine when I didn't work..."

I asked about access and he said he had to arrive at dawn to get a place.

"When Paidéia came, we did the training and then I began to understand things better. Then there was the reception, but even then there isn't a place for everyone... You know, right? Today I take the kids straight there and tell them to brush, but sometimes they forget. We have to stay on top of it.... They're older too, I'm not going to brush them anymore. I work all day, I come home tired, I make dinner, I wash the clothes, I have to keep an eye on whether they've done their homework... It's a lot and "M" [referring to her husband] doesn't help at all. He even plays video games with them..."

Finally, I ended by questioning why she never had a prosthesis made to rehabilitate the space she had lost. After all, she is now a CHA and works in a health center, and she knows about the importance of oral health in general health.

He replies that he never missed it. He says he always liked your smile and now he likes it even more. He asks if his picture will appear at work and says he'll "want to show it to everyone..." "Until you came to work here, I never went for it. It was only when you gave that presentation at the end of the year that I realized that missing teeth could cause other problems. Now I can see for myself, because even chewing is much better. "

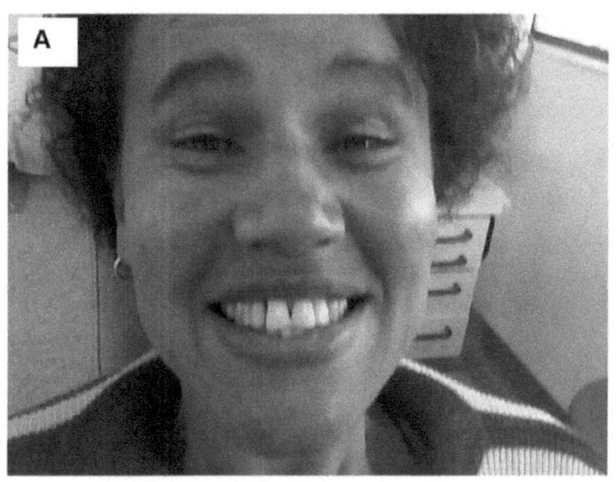

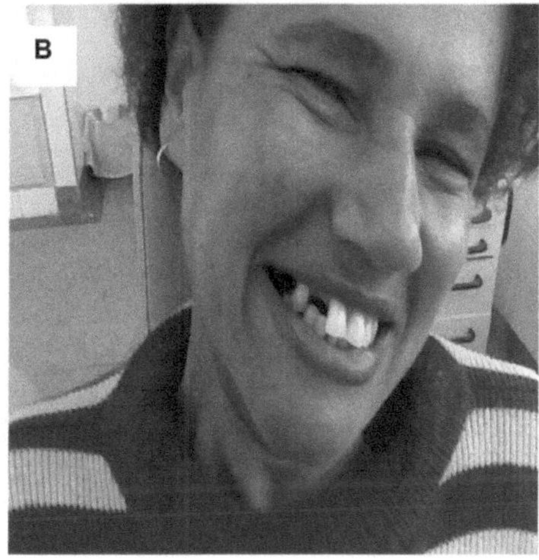

Image 4: Community health worker with a restored smile (A) and a very beautiful smile, even if "incomplete" (B)

6. "Chàcara Boy"

S.F.M. has lived on a farm in Joaquim Egidio, a district of Campinas, since she was born on June 1, 1987. She agreed to take part in the research as long as it was on the days she came to try out her prostheses, because the distance was too far to come on other days and her "boss" might not like us going there, because he might think we were getting in the way of his work. He spoke very little, but answered questions calmly and clearly.

His father was an employee of the same farm and had four other brothers. He was the second of five children. The owner was a nice man who had a lot of money, lived in the city [referring to Campinas] and went with his family on weekends to have fun. There was a swimming pool, barbecue area, three horses, a vegetable garden, a small corn and banana plantation. The owners used to bring friends and sometimes rented it out for parties or events.

He tells me that he and all his siblings were born there. His father didn't have a car, so he couldn't take his mother to the maternity hospital. But he says that his mother is a strong woman and helps out a lot at the weekends. She also helped when the children (the bosses' children) were small. They had a good life because their father was free to plant whatever he wanted and they lived in a house on the farm, but they didn't pay rent. In return, they had to keep the land and the swimming pool clean and the corn and bananas were sold at the re- dondezas so that "the farm wouldn't make a loss". They all studied until high school at the municipal school. They walked there early in the morning, came back, had lunch and had to help their father with the plantations. I asked if they didn't play and what time they did their schoolwork. He replied that they swam in the pool from time to time, rode horses, played hide and seek among themselves.

He says that only his middle brother has gone to the city to find work and is now working in a food store at the mall.

"He's the cashier, he handles a lot of money, but he has to account for it properly. He takes the orders and the people in the kitchen prepare them. But it's all frozen.... They just heat it up. He was also the only one who didn't get married. My two sisters got married and left. "R" [referring to his older brother] works on a farm further down the road, but we always meet up. We see the girls less..." I asked you how you lost your teeth and, since then, what has happened in your life?

"- The teeth kept getting damaged and one day it dawned this big [showing with his hands how big his face had become with the swelling], so there was no way, I had to go to the clinic. When I got there, I didn't even queue or anything, because the girl at the reception desk saw the look on my face and told me to go straight to the back, to the dentists. The dental lady told me that the doctor would have to give me medicine and then take it out. It was awful, because I had to take a really crazy injection and then I had to wait to get the tooth out, until my wife said it smelled bad and I couldn't escape... I had to go and get it out..."

I ask him why he puts things off and he says he's never liked dentists or that "little motor that seems to go into your soul". I realize how difficult it is to deal with fear, preferring even pain... And putting it off, whenever possible, until it's too late.

He also told me that after he had his teeth removed, he was very "upset" because he felt bad in front of his family, who said they didn't like it. "Nobody likes to look ugly, right? I've never been about beauty. It's a woman who has to be beautiful for us, but even my son said it was very ugly without the teeth". I went back to the clinic to see if the doctor could help and then she said she had you, that she could do it for several clinics and that I had to go. It was okay to take three buses, but it was cheaper than paying for a "perereca" in the city. My brother said it was around 500 dollars to go to a private dentist. I preferred to take the buses and come here."

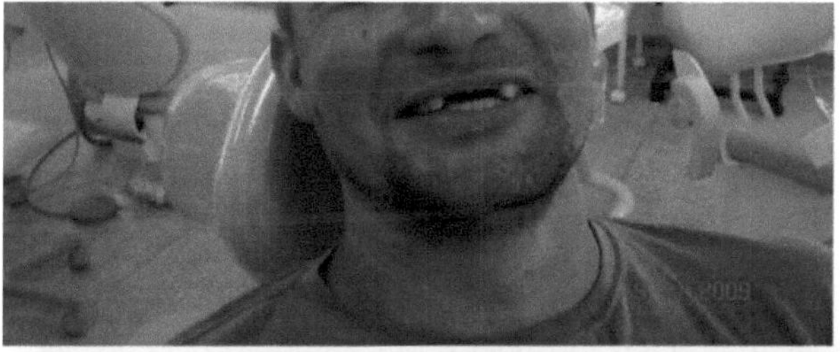
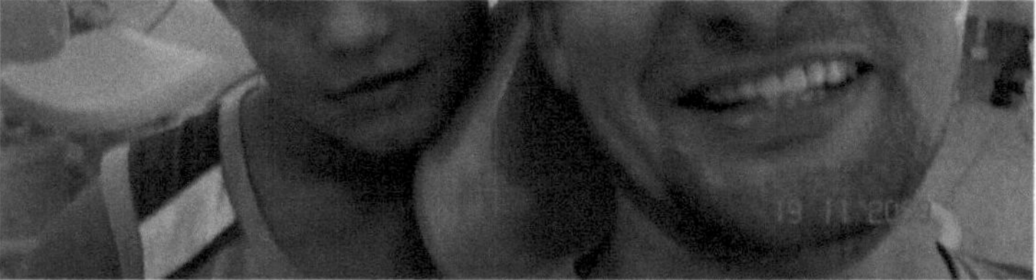

Image 5: "Moço da Châcara" proud and happy to show his son his rehabilitation.

7. "Lord of swollen feet"

I needed to interview a patient, if possible a man, over the age of 74 and who already had a prosthesis fitted, in order to complete the proposed table with gender and age equivalences. I took out my notebook and searched until I came across Mr.

J.R., born in 1934, phoned and was told by his wife that he was in hospital at Unicamp. I wrote down his room number and went to visit him at the Hospital de Clinicas (HC at Unicamp). When I arrived, I asked him if he remembered me and he promptly said that he would never forget the doctor who made his dentures. Surprised by my visit, he asked if I was working there and I replied that I was not. I just went to visit him. He seemed in a good mood, said he was very happy to see me and that he was honored by my visit. He immediately agreed to collaborate and answer questions, as soon as I explained why I had come to the hospital.

He had been hospitalized because his blood pressure and diabetes had decompensated. He told me that he took his medication "just right" [eleven tablets a day in total], but that it was very difficult to follow a diet and that he couldn't do any physical activity because his legs and feet swelled up too much. He was obese, had been on disability pension for several years and said he really liked watching soccer, drinking beer or "a branquinha", smoking and eating well. Everything that the doctors had forbidden him to do and that, as a result, life had lost its fun.

"Since I'm really going to die, at least I want to die happy. The woman hides all the good food from me and comes up with that unsalted rice and chayote... I can't stand it.... I remember that when the doctor put my teeth back in, all I could think about was eating a rib and gnawing on the little bones until the meat was gone...Uhnnn... Just saying that makes my mouth water..."

I talked to him, explaining that it was his excesses that had led him to that hospital bed and that he should try to follow the doctors' instructions, otherwise he would end up dying... He replies that he would rather die...

I try to distract him by changing the subject and ask him about his childhood, adolescence, his life before he became ill.

"Ahhhh... it was all very good. I grew up in the street, playing ball. In fact, even sock ball, because there was so much poverty and nobody had a good leather ball... but it was sock ball, it was old cans, bottle caps, anything we could kick and score was worth it... I was a happy kid in the sun and rain, shirtless, barefoot, with no time for anything. I only went home when my mother shouted my name, saying that dinner was ready".

I took advantage of the "cue" to talk about hygiene, and jokingly asked him if he had at least washed his hands for dinner? He laughs a lot and says:

"-Nothing to wash my hands with... I was so hungry that I'd go inside and eat whatever was in front of me..."

I ask him about brushing his teeth after a meal and he laughs heartily and says he didn't even know he had teeth...

The conversation progressed happily until a nursing assistant came in to check his blood pressure and take his temperature. He had no fever and his blood pressure was 140x110. It was still quite high and so he would remain in hospital for a while longer. After the nurse left the room, we resumed our conversation and I asked him how he had lost his teeth.

"Ahhh... I don't even remember, it's been so long... I pulled out some that got soft, others I went to the post office or to a clinic in town, I don't even remember anymore. I only remember one deep down that I pulled out in the city and it bled all night... it was the most difficult time I've ever been through... I even thought I was going to die... a towel was soaked in blood, it gave me a fever, my mouth swelled up, I couldn't even open it..."

I asked him why he didn't go to the dentist for prevention, so that his teeth wouldn't have to be extracted, but rather to look after them without having to remove them. He replied very calmly:

"- Ahhhh doctor... we were poor and poor people don't take care of their teeth, their health, anything. We just go on living, living life as God wants us to. We live just for the sake of living. You eat, work and sleep, that's all. We only go after things when the going gets tough, when the going gets tough. Can't you see that I'm here in this bed? I had to get very sick, I had chills, pain in my chest, in my head, I saw everything dark, then the woman thought I was going to die and called SAMU. The SAMU went there, measured my blood pressure and said it was 21 over 15 and brought me here with the siren on and everything. I think even they thought I was going to die... But bad things don't die, do they?" [he says with a tense smile on his face].

We talked some more and I tried to cheer him up, to joke around. The atmosphere became heavy. There was a sadness in the air ....

I left with a bad feeling, of unease and sadness. What would become of him????

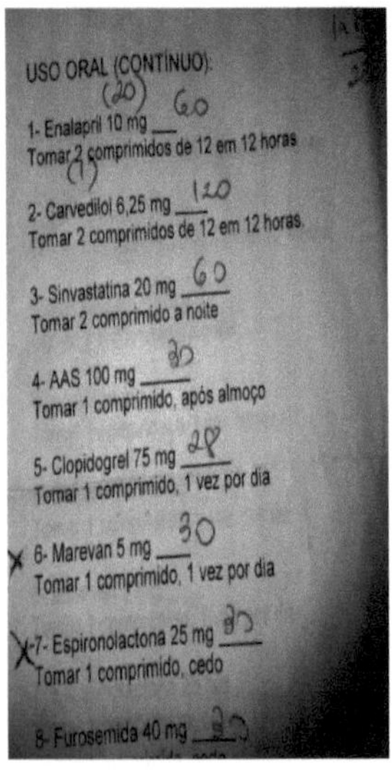

Image 6: Some of the medicines taken by "Mr. Inchy Feet"

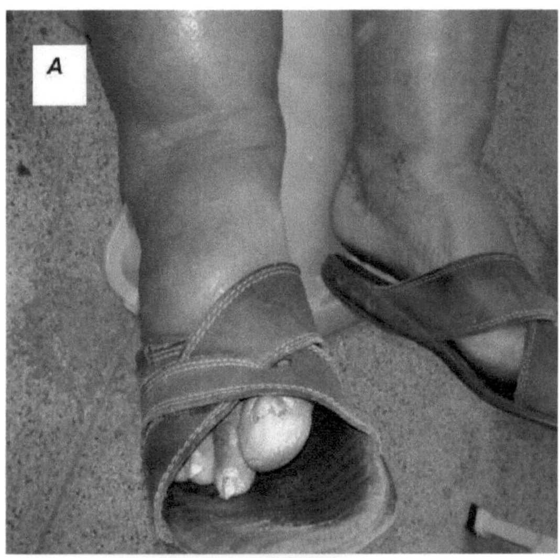

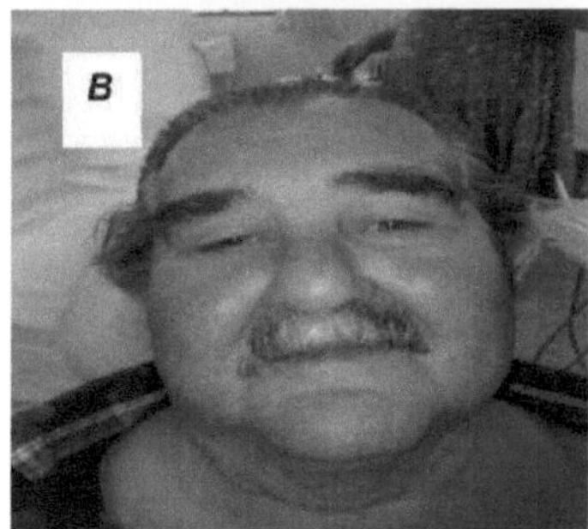

Image 7: In "A" the photograph taken of her feet when she was making her prostheses and was already undergoing clinical treatment for hypertension and diabetes. And in "B" the face of sadness at the impossibility, due to illness, of doing everything she liked in life: eating, drinking and
smoking.

8. "Mrs. Warrior"

A 63-year-old patient, very lucid, despite having had five strokes, active, talkative, made a point of taking part in the work and welcoming us into her home. It was a very pleasant Saturday afternoon, with coffee and creamy cornmeal cake with guava.

He tells me about his difficult childhood in Minas Gerais, on a farm, with four other siblings, a mother, a father and a grandmother who lived together. There weren't many resources, no television, they played climbing trees, ciranda, and rode horses. When they got older, they started helping their parents with the coffee plantations. She only learned to read at the age of 50 because she married a boy from Minas when she was 17 and came to live in Campinas. "He got a job at Pirelli and I came with him. I had my three children and I just looked after them and the house. I became a widow at the age of 30 and then I had to work to finish raising the children. That's when I realized I needed to learn to read. Because until then I had never felt the need. But how? I couldn't go to school at my age. I learned a lot later with a very generous boss who taught me. One day I took a tumble in the bathroom and lost 14 teeth in one go. I think it was because of the stroke. You remember, don't you? I've already told you that I've had five strokes... and here I am, like a rock. I take those 14 medicines a day, I don't eat anything with salt and I go for walks, everything the doctors tell me to. "

When I asked her how she looked after her teeth, she smiled and said that her teeth were her treasure. "In Minas Gerais we didn't have a toothbrush, but my grandmother used to pick a bush, a climbing plant, and we used it to take a bath, scrub our whole body and our teeth too. It was better than these brushes sold in the markets. It cleans very well."

When I ask him about the prostheses, the service and the stages of molding, fitting and delivery, he smiles and says: "My daughter, for someone who has had to fight so much in this life, these bridges fell out of the sky. I didn't even know that post offices made bridges. I only found out because I used to go there so much to measure my blood pressure, one day I saw you, with your friendliness, talking to a man and explaining to him that if it hurt, he could come back at any time. I got curious and asked the nurse, and she told me that you made dentures and that you had to put your name on the list because it took a long time to get through. I went there and gave my name. It took three or four years to be called, but I was a widow, so there was no problem. For me, what was worse than the years I waited was seeing her agonize every time she had to try it. It went wrong a couple of times, didn't it? You always apologized, explained to me the problem with the laboratory that was far away, but you got nervous when it didn't work out. Now I'm gorgeous! I go to bingo, to the SESI ball, I do my group walks and everyone says I look better. Now you need to take more care of yourself and not be so nervous, right? Leave the others behind and do your job with the love you have. God sees everything, my child".

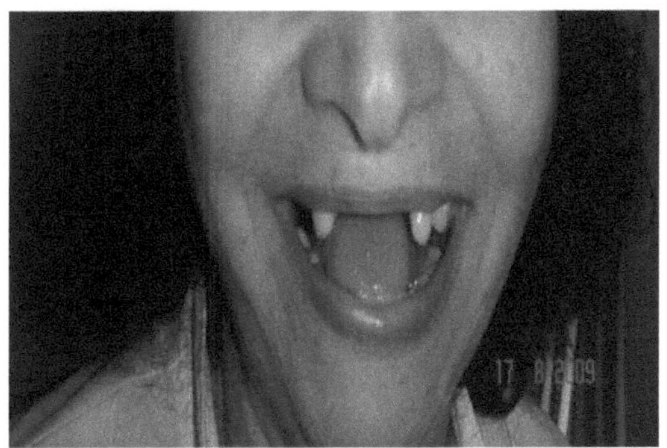

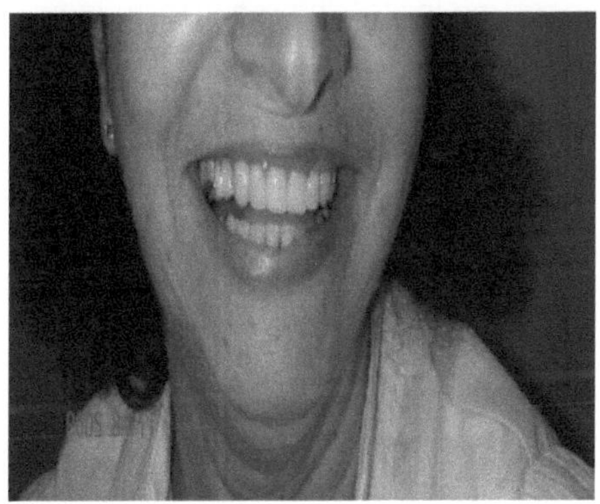

Image 8: "Mrs. Guerreira, before (A) and after (B) the Removable Partial Prosthesis, a rescue for oral health and self-esteem.

9. *"Young believer"*

He was born on February 24, 1965 in the interior of Paranà and moved to Campinas as a boy. He comes from a family of 8 siblings, father and mother already deceased, married, no children. He works as a bricklayer or painter and says that he "takes any job that comes along... If God provides and blesses, I do it and I do it well, whatever it is..."

He came with an "URGENCY" referral, with no vacancies allocated by the district, knocked on the door and was very anxious. I remember he spoke very quickly and was a little confused, but I asked him to calm down and he explained himself better:

"- Doctor "R" [Dentist at the Sâo Quirino Health Center] had to take out my teeth because they had softened and she said there was no repair. Now I have nothing, but I can't stay like this because I'm going to be a pastor, I really want to be a pastor, I know this is the path the Lord has prepared for me, and I can't run away, but how am I going to be a pastor without my teeth? How am I going to go to the pulpit and preach without my teeth? I really need my teeth and Doctor "R" explained that there's a long queue, that it could take many years to call me, but I can't wait all that, I really need my teeth... you have to find a way, they said that only you can find a way..."

I ended up fitting it in and everything worked out! The service went very smoothly. There were no delays, no changes, no losses, no repetitions. In two months he had his full dentures ready. He never missed any appointments or arrived late. Every time he entered the room, he blessed me and thanked me. When he left, the procedure was the same: blessings and thanks.

For all these reasons, it was a case that stood out to me and as soon as I had to select cases for interviews, I immediately remembered to call him.

He was very happy to see me and offered to give me an appointment at the health center itself, so that I wouldn't have to drive all the way to his house, claiming it was far away...

Since he was a child, he always went to church with his parents and grew up saying he was going to be a pastor. He says that he had a very "rough" upbringing and that his father used to beat him and his brothers with a stick when they did something...

Everyone sat at the table together for meals and there was no television at home, so after homework they would read the Bible and go to bed.

"We were very poor, but the church never let us lack anything. They even gave us food parcels so we could eat. My father worked as a bricklayer and at the church he did everything they needed. He repaired chairs, replaced roof tiles, or anything else that was needed, which is why they also took such good care of our family. "

I asked her about hygiene and she quickly said that her mother was very clean and demanded that her children were too. They didn't always have water in the tap, so her mother would fetch it from a well with a can and bathe them with a mug. "There was only one toothbrush to clean their teeth, but she told them to do it and they all did it," she said proudly. "You can ask doctor "R" [referring to the dentist who had made the referral], my teeth were all very white and brushed, but I got gum disease and they became very soft... that's why I had to have them pulled out."

Daily of 08/02/2017

Today I saw a man who was having an outburst. He came with a referral from Sao Quirino [one of the UBSs that refer patients for prostheses]. I tried my best to explain that everyone who has their teeth removed, for one reason or another, needs to have them replaced, but there is only one professional to make the prostheses for all 10 units in the city's Eastern District. It was no use, the man was out of control and talking non-stop. He prayed, talked to himself, turned to me, looked up, begged, pleaded... I ended up giving in. I know I shouldn't fit in, but I feel sorry for him... it seems like I'm the one who doesn't want to... But why do they make the referral and then knock on my door? At Sao Quirino, they should just say there's no vacancy and that's that. Let them put him on the waiting list there and not tell him to come here and talk to me.

"C"] came to talk to me and that ladainha I already know. You can't fit everyone in... If every person who comes here grumbling, whining, asking, you fit them in, your schedule becomes like this, with no conditions... I know, but it's hard to be the one to say "NO". In the end, I just give up!

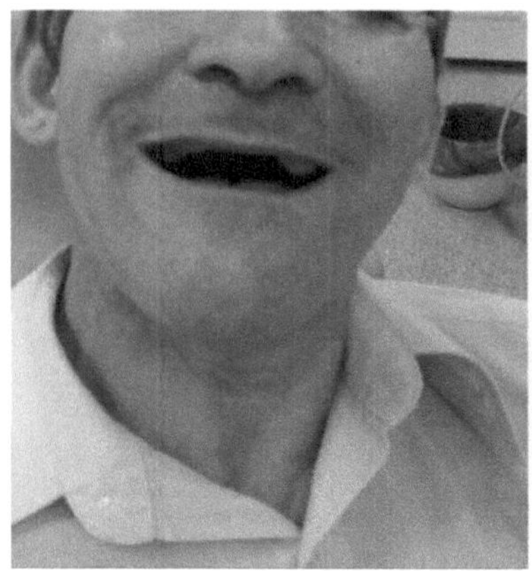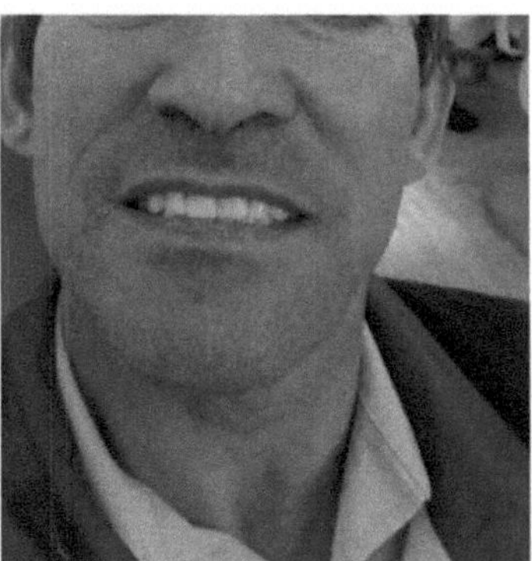

Image 9: "Young believer" who needed his teeth to be able to climb the pulpit and fulfill his dream of becoming a pastor.

10. "Cancer boy"

Dr. "D" [a colleague who works with me at the Health Center] came to talk to me about a patient he had seen at Unicamp who had to have all his teeth extracted because he had throat cancer. After surgical removal, he had to undergo chemotherapy and radiotherapy. The Unicamp protocol recommends total extraction in these cases to prevent radioosteonecrosis[14] posteriorly. As a result, the patient became totally edentulous and was very depressed. We agreed that I would fit him in.

On the scheduled day, the patient appeared very downcast, with a sad look on his face and a very unhealthy appearance...

We got talking and I encouraged him to tell his story. He was married, had two daughters, a small printing company in his own home and had been a smoker for many years, which had contributed to his throat cancer. He spoke very quietly due to the recent surgery, as he was still in pain, but it was also clear that his tone was low due to melancholy.

I molded the ridge, made and adjusted the prostheses and when I finished, it was clear that my self-esteem had returned. Throughout the treatment we formed bonds of affection and friendship. He was still a very vain gentleman

---

*14 **Radioosteonecrosis** is one of the most serious complications of radiotherapy used to treat head and neck cancer.*

who was more bothered by the absence of his teeth than by the disease itself.

Three years after the installation of the two total prostheses, I contacted him to invite him to take part in the research. He readily accepted and preferred to go to the Health Center to see Dr. "D" and me and to take the opportunity to answer the interview questions.

When he met us, he showed great joy and satisfaction. She brought chocolates for the entire dental team and special gifts for me and Dr. "D".

We sat down and talked. His illness had stalled. I had regular check-ups at Unicamp and everything led me to believe that I would be cured if my condition remained the same for the next two years.

He told me that adapting to the prostheses was much easier than he had imagined. "It was really hard to stop smoking... sometimes I still find myself putting my hand in my pocket to get the packet. "

He answered questions very clearly and quickly. It seemed that the subject she most wanted to talk about was her current health situation. Having been so frightened by the cancer diagnosis and now feeling that it's all behind her was very encouraging.

She had a happy childhood, although her parents were divorced. She said she liked her stepfather and even preferred him to her father, because the latter sometimes beat her mother. "We were little, but I remember the fights and my mother screaming when he hit her. Then, after a while, he got together with my stepfather, who was also separated and had three other children. Today we're all friends.

When I asked her about her health, how she took care of it, who took care of it, she immediately referred to her teeth and said that it was her mother who told her to brush them and if any of them hurt or were damaged, they would go to the clinic to get a place with a dentist.

I asked why I was going to get a parking space at dawn and the answer was immediate:

"- ahhh... you either went at dawn or you didn't get in. There were few vacancies, so you had to go early. "

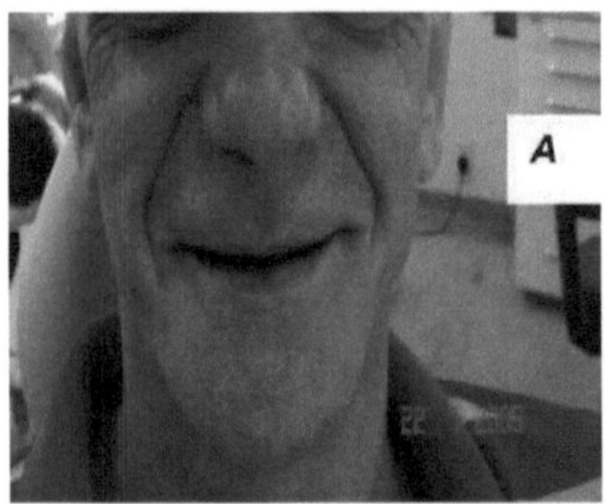

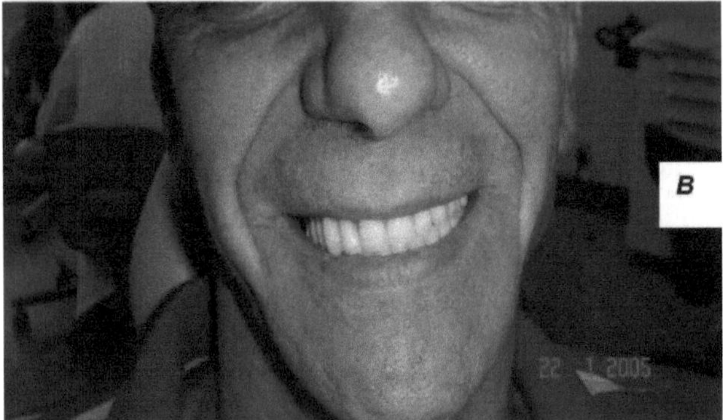

Image 10: The need for chemo- and radiotherapy meant that all the teeth had to be extracted (A) and after rehabilitation, self-esteem, which had been totally shattered, was restored (B).

11. *"Mrs. Toothless"*

She was born right here in Campinas, on August 14, 1992. She came to the Health Center after being referred by one of our referral units. I've never forgotten the look on that girl's face when she walked into my office and immediately said: "Doctor, tell me you're going to help me..." And then she started crying... I asked her to come in, sit down and calm down so we could talk. She began by saying that she'd been to the dentist all her life and no one had ever solved her problem. She said that she'd always taken care of herself and done everything she'd been told, but she'd always ended up "taking her teeth out"... and that now it was her front teeth, which made her husband say he wouldn't look at her anymore...

It was a very interesting case that I will always remember. When we set up the doctoral project and decided that we would interview three groups of patients (the "waiting list" group, the group of patients undergoing treatment and the group of people who had already completed their prostheses), I immediately remembered her and wanted to interview her. I really wanted to hear from her, how she was doing and whether she had adapted well to her prostheses.

I looked up Mrs. Banguela's phone number in my prosthesis notebook, called her to talk about my doctorate and see if she would agree to be interviewed, and she answered. She recognized my voice right away! She said she missed me. I explained everything and she agreed on the spot. We met right here at the station. She said she'd like to see me and I'd like to see her with her dentures and her teeth brushed. She said she was taking very good care of them.

In the interview, she told me that she was the daughter of a single mother and that she had two other brothers, one from each father. They all lived in her grandmother's house and the two older brothers helped make the food, wash the clothes and do the cleaning, because her grandmother was very ill. So she took care of her own health, schoolwork, personal hygiene and food. When I asked her about her mother, she said that she worked all day, in a family home, and when she got home she was always very tired and just wanted to watch TV and sleep. However, she says with certainty that she took very good care of herself: "I always liked to shower and smell good... I didn't have soap or fancy shampoo, but I had one there that was enough. I also brushed all my teeth. " She says: "... when a tooth was cracked or hurting, my brothers would take me to the post office, but there they'd remove the hole and put a paste on it, or they'd pull it out." When I ask her about a memorable event, she remembers a time when she had a tooth extracted and bled all night. She talks about it smiling, joking, as if it didn't matter much, on the contrary, as if it was something normal...

She finally married a good man, had two daughters and says she's very happy. "The problem was just my teeth, doctor. My life is good! I have my little house, my daughters, my husband's work is good... But when my front teeth got soft and that dentist at my clinic said I was going to have to have them pulled, and I came home and told my husband I was going to be lame, he immediately said he wasn't even going to look me in the face You can see that you remember that my teeth were fine, right? They didn't even have holes in them, they weren't black... It's just that my teeth are always like that... They get soft. But thank God God put you in my life and told me I wouldn't have my teeth out until the bridge was ready. And it all worked out, don't you remember? Today I don't even look like I'm wearing a bridge. Everyone says my teeth are beautiful. But the best thing was the way you taught me to brush my teeth. I don't understand why no one ever told me that I also had to brush my gums and that this was what made my teeth soft... Now we all brush like this at home. The girls have learned how to make balls and massage the ginger. I'll tell you something. Now that I no longer have that smell in my mouth, my husband gives me those good kisses... on the mouth!!! It's true! After I put my teeth in, my husband even started kissing me again..."

Daily of 23/03/2013

Today I delivered Mrs. Banguela's prostheses. It was a really nice case, I don't think I'll ever forget it. ....The dentures weren't that good, but she was so happy! To think they were going to take her teeth out and leave her completely without front teeth Sometimes I wonder why dentists are so lazy. What does it cost to teach someone to brush their teeth? How much time is wasted? If someone had ever taught this girl to brush her teeth, I doubt she would have lost her teeth. But no, extraction is easier. Saying that she has periodontal disease, that she's a pig, that she doesn't brush properly, that she doesn't floss, is easy. Don't they think that a tube of dental floss costs about 6 reais? Don't they think that sometimes people don't even have enough money to eat, so how are they going to spend on floss? Why don't they offer alternatives? Why don't they say that it's possible to exchange dental floss for sewing thread or kite string? Why don't they interact with the patient? Don't they talk, ask questions? Don't you listen?

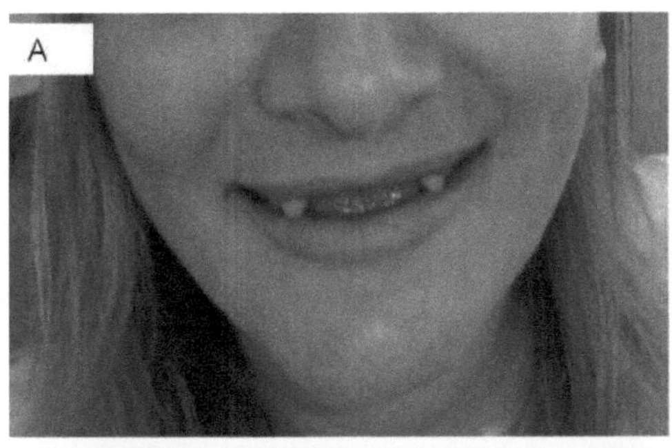

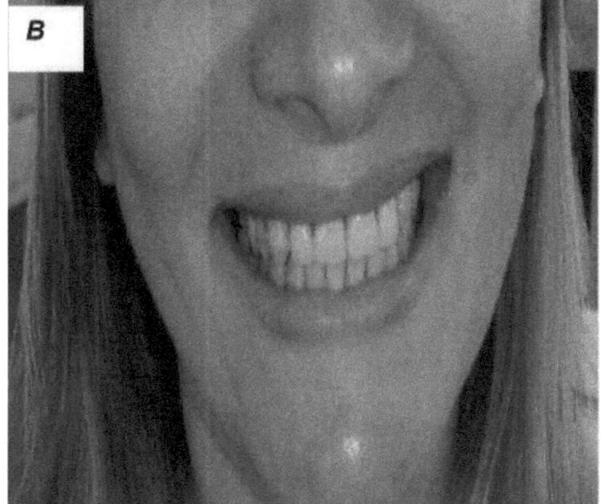

Image 11: "Mrs. Banguela in (A) without the anterior dental elements and in (B) after the recovery of her mouth with the use of prostheses.

12. "Cashier girl"

A 22-year-old girl who doesn't like to talk much, but agrees to take part in the survey. She answers the questions all the time with her hands in front of her mouth. She carries with her the pain and shame of having lost her teeth. She smiles shyly when I tell her that she can take her hand away from her mouth because now she has teeth and she looks beautiful! She says that the best thing in her life was getting the bridge and being hired as a cashier at the hypermarket. It was a very quick interview because she just answered the questions bluntly, directly. She told me that she was born right here in the city and still lived with her parents. She studied until she finished high school and then went to work in order to earn money and contribute to the household expenses. Her teeth were already decayed and when she went to the health

103

center to have them restored, they told her that the canals would have to be treated. "As it didn't hurt, I left it alone, until one day I decided to go to the health center to get it fixed. The dentists said I had to have a root canal and that there was a waiting list of about two years... so I waited, but my turn never came. One day it got swollen and I went to the clinic and they said I had to pay privately to have the canals done or have them pulled. I didn't have a choice, did I? So I pulled it out..."

Daily of 23/07/2012

I received a referral from the Sâo Quirino Health Center with an "urgency" stamp. She was a girl with no front teeth who needed to have them fitted in order to get a job at (the name of a well-known hypermarket). She'd had an interview and the manager told her that he couldn't hire her unless she put in her missing teeth. We really do live in a country of absurditiesIf the girl doesn't have teeth, it's obviously because she doesn't have the money to put them in, and if she doesn't get a job because of this, how is she going to do it? I'm glad there are still people with enough common sense and sensitivity to realize such a need. I'm reminded of "Dr. Augustinho" and the barbaric things he did: anesthetize a patient and send him back in the afternoon just because he wanted to leave soon and that gentleman came in dying of pain right at the end of his period... or worse, the

the day he told the little man that he had to brush his teeth better, because that pain was because he wasn't brushing properly. He also signed and stamped the medical record after noting that there was a need to improve hygiene conditions. ....We saw the patient in the afternoon, because, of course, he came back in pain, saying that he had brushed a lot, but the pain never got better... and "M" (the name of a fellow dentist) extracted the two little teeth with his hand, because they were so mobile Would it have hurt to give him some pain medication?

Would it hurt to explain that there was a disease and that those teeth were lost and would have to be extracted? I don't know who's worse... "Augustinho", who just wants to "break his hand" and collect his salary from the town hall at the end of the month, or the coordinator, the supporter, in short, the boss, the manager who knows everything and does nothing because he's "permanent"? It's tough!!!!

But at least we have the consolation of having people who are people, human, responsible, involved and sensitive enough to realize that the girl needs her teeth to get the job, like Doctor "C" from Sâo Quirino.

At this point in her life, that's what she needs, her teeth... And we're going to get dentures, of course!!!

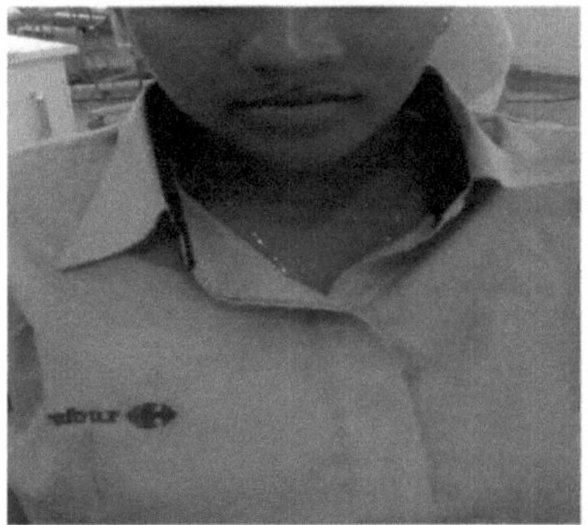

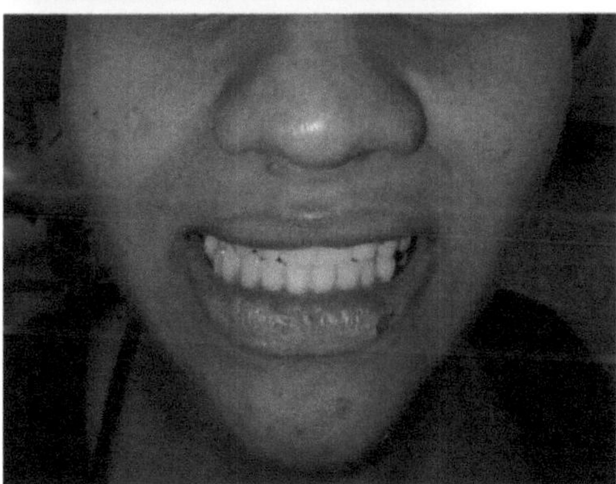

Image 12: "Cashier girl" who had to get her teeth done in order to be hired to work at the hypermarket checkout.

13. "Little Stroke Lady"

We phoned a lady who had been on the waiting list for almost three years and talked to her daughter "K" about the possibility of interviewing her for a research project. At first she wasn't very receptive and tried to shy away, but as we explained the importance of using the work as a "wake-up call" about the difficulty of accessing the service and the delay in summoning people, like her mother, to be called for prostheses, she changed her mind and agreed to see us. We went on the day and at the time arranged by "K". It was a very simple house in a nearby neighborhood, attached to the Costa e Silva Health Center.

We were welcomed and invited to enter and sit down in the room where the "little lady with the stroke" was already sitting. Very thin and haggard, sitting on a wheelchair, we realized that she was lucid, but with very limited movement.

The daughter immediately said:

"- At last they're going to make the dentures, in a few minutes Mom would have died and you wouldn't have called yet.... I had the SAD [Home Care] staff pull out the last teeth she had left because they were so badly damaged, but that was a long time ago.... They said they would put her name on the waiting list, but it took too long..."

I explained that we weren't there to make the prosthesis, but for an assessment and a chat, with the possibility of recording, if she agreed, for research purposes. Mrs. K became very irritated and said that we could record her, but that she was going to "stick her mouth in" ... "Where have you seen that?" she asked. In her view, rehabilitating her mother with prostheses would be a benefit, as it would make it easier for her to eat. There would be no more need to make soups or min- gau, because her mother would be able to eat the food that everyone in the house ate. She explained that it was very difficult to keep her mother "in this state" and that the other siblings didn't want to share the responsibility. "It's all left to me," she said, complaining about the work she now had to do with baths, changing diapers, eating different foods than she did for the other members of the family, and the cost of diapers and medicines that the Health Center didn't provide.

I understood the degree of difficulty her mother's current state of health was causing her and her anxiety about having the prostheses fitted, but I explained the difficulties inherent in the case. With muscle limitations and atrophy of the facial nerves, it would be very difficult to fit prostheses, especially the lower one, and chewing would be very difficult, so there was no indication for such a diagnosis.

At the end of the conversation, many questions were clarified, but I was left without the answers to the survey. "K" couldn't tell us about her mother's oral health care during the various stages of her life and the "little lady", although lucid, found it very difficult to speak. We could tell from her smiles, eye movements and expressions that she understood everything that was being discussed.

When we said goodbye, we realized that the little lady had been relieved, but "K", who was already very stressed, was even more so. She complained a lot and asked several times if we were recording what she was saying... "I wanted my indignation with this town hall to be well recorded."

Daily of 11/10/2013[15]

Today I saw a lady who had had a stroke and was left with various symptoms. She can no longer walk, hardly moves her arms and has great difficulty speaking. Her daughter told me that she "had" her teeth pulled out because they were ugly and damaged... I had to take a deep breath as I listened to the story, and an even deeper one to explain that rehabilitating this lady with two total prostheses was not the solution; on the contrary, it would be an additional inconvenience (...). At the end of the conversation, the little lady, with a lot of effort, gave a big smile and thanked me. In fact, this was not her wish, but her daughter's. I was happy, despite the daughter's complaints, who only mentioned us [she was accompanied by an assistant] and the town hall. She badmouthed everything. The government, politicians, corruption... Her problem, poor thing, was having to take on the whole burden of looking after a sick mother and that alone was too much.... It can't be easy to change your whole life and have to structure yourself to look after your mother. God forbid... I hope my parents still have a lot of health ahead of them.

---

15 This diary is of a very similar case to the pathological story of the "Little Lady with the Stroke", which is why it has been posted here. The stories are sometimes very similar...

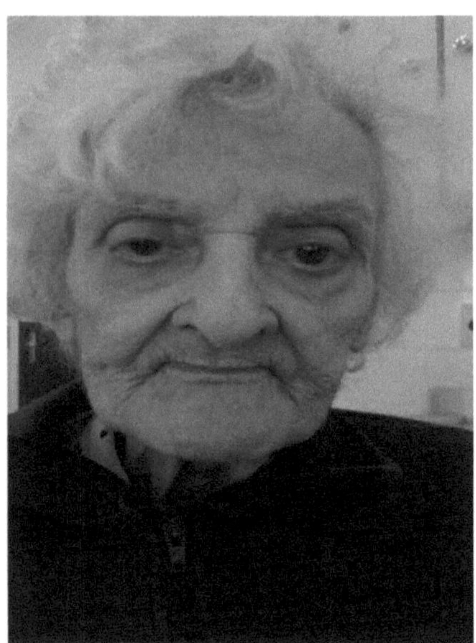

Image 13: "Little Stroke Lady"

14. "Ponte Preta fan"

M. C. R., the symbolic Ponte Preta fan, is a 78-year-old woman who lives in a small apartment in a popular neighborhood of the city, known by the Health Center and by the whole neighborhood for her "fanaticism" about her soccer team. She was born in Casa Branca, the daughter of a woman who was hospitalized in an old sanatorium in Cocais and died shortly after giving birth. She never knew her parents and went to an orphanage where she left to work and live with a family from Carapicuiba.

The girl was only 12 when she moved to Campinas to live with Mrs. Ivone. It was Paulinho, her boss's son, who accompanied her to a match at the "Majestic Ponte Preta Stadium". Since then, she has frequented the stands and has always been highly respected, she says. Her attachment to the team from Campinas began around 1950, when the stadium was built. "I was very curious to see inside, what it was like... so I went. I was impressed! People said how beautiful it was... ....We watched the match, I don't even remember

which one. I just remember the fans shouting, cheering, vibrating... the stands even seemed to shake. Now I watch most of the games on television, but because of my fanaticism for the soccer team, I became very well known and popular with the Ponte Pretana fans. " On the days of decisive matches, some friends get together and take her on their laps to go down the stairs from the apartment (there is no elevator in the building) and take her to the stadium.

She suffered an ischemic stroke when she was almost 40 and was taken in at the PUC hospital where she had an acquaintance of Mrs. Ivone's who worked in external relations and who found a way to fit her in ...

Today, more than 30 years later, she is bedridden and receives visits from the Health Center, the doctor, the physiotherapy team and the nursing staff. "The dentist never came," she says. "Only now, because my name has been on the waiting list for dentures for four years..."

A very active, smiling, cheerful and talkative person who doesn't seem to be saddened by the situation she finds herself in. She wakes up every day at around nine o'clock in the morning and takes her "pretinho". "I won't stay without it. Then I light my cigarette and listen to the radio until lunchtime. Sometimes the people from the health center come to examine me or do some exercise. After lunch I always take a nap and in the evening I like to watch soap operas. I watch them all until I go to sleep. Now, if there's a match on, I don't miss it!!! I light up! I've always liked it. My boss, D. Iolanda, was rich and lived in a huge house in Castelo, but even I convinced her to go to the match with me. She was all chic in the middle of the crowd! Can you?"

Not many people know, but she was married to a Guarani fan (a rival team from the same city). When we talk about it, the mood changes. She closes her smile and says: "The only good thing about him is the house he left me and the pension I receive. "

He lights one cigarette after another and says it's his companion for all hours. "Yes, referring to the cigarette, although all the doctors say I have to 'give up' the habit..."

She tells us that she took her teeth out as they got damaged and at the clinic they thought it was better to pull them out because there was no way of fixing them.... She is now totally edentulous and remains on the waiting list for prostheses, although she already has a very old upper prosthesis, but it is in good condition.

The only complaint he had was paresthesia in the right corner of his mouth, due to the sequelae of the ischemic stroke, but he says he's already taking B-complex and will soon get better, God willing.

While we were talking, she asked if it was past midday and when we asked her why, she said she was hungry and the "marmitex" was taking too long to arrive... She says that there's a girl who comes once a week to clean the house and wash the clothes, but she prefers to get the "marmitex" every day because it's always fresh. She only uses her very old dentures to go out. She says she chews everything with her gums, and has got used to it since she lost her teeth. She doesn't brush any more because she doesn't have any teeth, but she does rinse her teeth after lunch and dinner to "get rid of the debris that sticks to her mouth and soaks her dentures in water and vinegar to keep them well disinfected. "

Daily of January 10, 2017

Today we went to interview a bedridden woman who has been on the waiting list for total prostheses for over two years. Everyone at the health center knows her. They said I'd love to! It would be a lot of "stuff to talk about"... and it was! A lady who has suffered so much, with so many misfortunes throughout her life, but who smiles all the time. How could she? And we're complaining about so little... The mother died in childbirth and the father, unknown, was also an inmate at a clinic for the mentally ill in Casa Branca. There was no paternal name or surname in the family file. She was adopted at the age of 12 by a family who gave her bed and board in exchange for housework, but even so, she says she is very grateful to God and to D. Ivone who brought her up and even "allowed" her to go to school to learn how to read and write...My goodness, how can she?

So much complacency in one person.... When we told her that we weren't going to make the prosthesis for the time being, because it wasn't her turn on the waiting list yet, she smiled and said it was fine. "I'm already very happy to have met you... and this one is still good enough..." [showing the old prosthesis in his mouth].

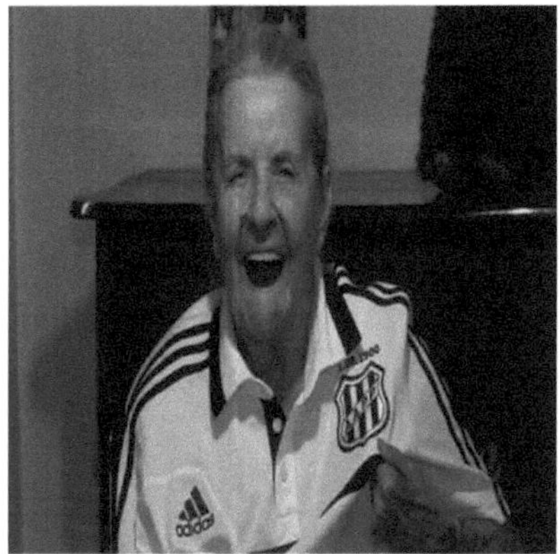

Image 14: Dona Conceiçao in the golden days of Ponte Preta (Reproduction of report 02/05/2017 VTV/SBT).

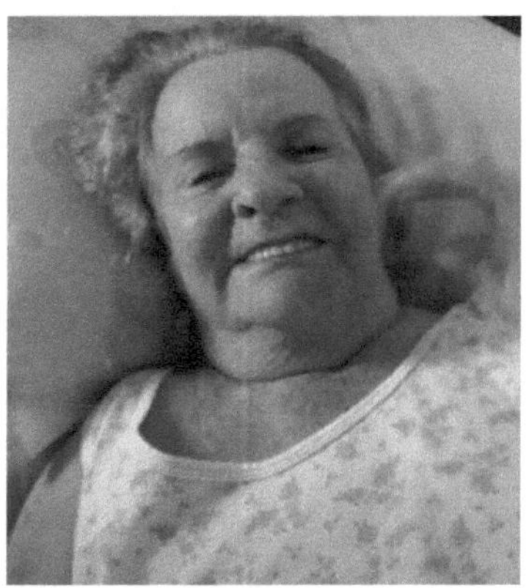

Image 15: Dona Conceiçao on the day of the interview

15. "Mr. Talking"

This pathological story comes from the northwest region of the city. As I've already mentioned in my implications, I'm also a lecturer at the PUC, which is located in the North-West District, and I make home visits with students where I end up coming across very unusual cases, such as this one. So we decided to include him in the research, even though he wasn't a user from the Eastern region (like everyone else), because he presented himself as a very interesting story.

A nursing assistant, "E", came to talk to us and said that we needed to visit "Mr. Talking", a patient who lived near the Ipaussurama Health Center, where PUC students do their internship. He told us that he had very few teeth in his mouth and complained of pain in one of them. I asked her to tell me a little about his history and she said that he had been shot when he was little and had little movement in his legs and arms, as well as losing sight in one eye. He already receives home visits from the team doctor, the physiotherapist from PUC and that they all know him well because he has lived there since the Health Center opened. He also says that he won't say any more because he loves telling his own story.

We only crossed the street because the house is right in front of the CS and there was a large open porch. There was a tiled roof and a yellow plastic table, one of those pub tables with a beer slogan on it, and several chairs around it. A gentleman was sitting on one of them with both arms resting on the table. His gaze was attentive to our arrival. Right next to him, a lady, a girl and a child holding a bag of fresh bread in one hand and a small loaf in the other, which they were enjoying with great pleasure. She offers one of the buns to the man and he takes it with great difficulty. We then realized that it was our patient. We said "good afternoon" and asked to be allowed to sit down. Quickly, the girl went to find some other chairs that were stacked in the corner and put them around the table so that there would be room for me and the four students accompanying me. I introduced myself and told him that I'd come to find out about his aching tooth, but first I wanted him to tell me a little bit about his story. He begins by introducing his little niece and ordering her to offer us the bread. The child readily obeys, but we say "no, thank you". He then asks if I'm new at the post, because he's never seen me before and says he knows everyone. I explained that I'm a professor at PUC and that's why I only go to the Health Center occasionally, but as I'm a referral for the prosthesis service, the assistant asked me to see if there was any possibility of making prostheses for him, in case he had to have that painful tooth extracted? He smiles and begins to tell his story.

He came from a family of 15 brothers who lived in the interior of Minas Gerais where their father had a farm. One day, they were on the balcony and a stray shot hit him in the head. I asked him how old he was and he said he was nine. He was taken to hospital, but as there were no resources, he was transferred to another, larger hospital near the capital, Belo Horizonte. He stayed there for over a year. His mother and older brothers took turns visiting him sporadically throughout this period. He says that he was left with many sequelae because "his nerves shrank and he could no longer stretch his legs and arms". She also lost her sight on her right side and shows it with difficulty, covering her left eye, which can't see us, only the other eye. They decided to sell the farm and come to Campinas. They bought the house where we were talking and said that: "...there was nothing here, not even the post office. There was only scrubland. So my father set up a bar to serve the truck drivers who passed through here and I helped out in the bar. When my father died, my mother continued with the bar and I always helped her. A lot of truck drivers used to come here from other towns. My brothers and sisters went to school, but it was far away for me, because with the nerves in my legs shrunk, I can't walk very far, so I didn't go. I only learned to read after many years when Mobral came to this area". When his mother died, he left his guardianship to his older sister, who received a pension to take care of him. But she got married and moved away, and ended up coming only sporadically to make lunch and do some of the housework. "She would come and feed me, brush my teeth and leave. Then my sister next door asked the social worker to take over my guardianship because she lives next door and has always looked after me. She and my nieces are always here (points to the lady, the girl and the child with the bag of bread)". She goes on to tell us about her life. He shows the PVC pipe handrail that his brother-in-law made so that he could support himself from the back, where the house used to be, to the front, where there was a tiled roof and a small door where the bar was. He also said that he liked to stand out front because he was closer to everyone, he could see the street, talk to the neighbors, help out in the bar (when he was younger) and watch the traffic... "I didn't like being stuck in there, at the back, without seeing anyone." In the course of the conversation, he shows the scars from the many surgeries he had undergone to try to regain movement. He tells us that it was he who gave the tip to "the physiotherapy doctor" when the Health Center had to move and there was no place to go. He was the one who showed her the land on which the Health Center was built and now stands. He also says that he knows all the doctors and has even been to one of them to see why he gets a toothache when he eats something sweet. I examine and notice a cavity, but the other elements are still well integrated, which will allow us to make two removable prostheses, after proper restoration of the tooth in question and a scraping (cleaning of tartar).

I have arranged with the sister who is there that I will make an appointment with the dentist at the Health Center to carry out the clinical procedures and then return with the students to take the molds for the prostheses in their own home.

Asked by her sister why this possibility of rehabilitation with prostheses was only available at this time, I explained that the prosthesis service works as a specialty in the municipality of Campinas. In other words, they aren't available in all the units as suggested by the Ministry of Health and this ends up generating a lot of demand which is "repressed" on a waiting list. Since this home visit took place, priority would be given to making the prostheses in the home itself, with an academic/didactic function for the students of the PUC School of Dentistry. The sister was grateful for the opportunity, but said that if there was a service, it wasn't fair that it should be for only a few: "They should give everyone who doesn't have a tooth a chance. My brother is more needy than me, but I had to pay to get my dentures... I've been on this list for over three years and I've never been called up... The right thing would be for everyone to win. Everyone who needs it because it's very expensive and we can't afford it, but we can't go without teeth either... How do we eat? How do you talk to other people if you don't have a tooth? It's very embarrassing because it seems like we're slackers and don't take care of ourselves, but we want to, but there's no room at the health center and so we pay to have our teeth pulled at the center and have them plated there... ".

A few weeks later, "Mr. Talking" is taken by his sister to the Health Center to have the aching tooth restored, and the assistant calls me to say that we can start making the prostheses. I set a date for another home visit, this time to take the first impression, and ask three students to accompany me.

We made the prostheses and, of course, made the patient very happy, but his sister remained angry. At every visit we made to take the molds and try them on, she reaffirmed her indignation. "Such a simple thing that you can do at home, why can't you do it for everyone? Politicians should be poor to see what it's like not to have teeth... Only those who don't have teeth know what we go through..."

Daily of 14/04/2017

Today I went to a house opposite the C.S. to do a home visit with the students. We talked to a little man who was shot when he was 9 years old. He's completely scarred, but happy. I even said this to the students. We're so privileged, we have everything and every now and then we're complaining about life... meanwhile, people who have nothing always seem to be enjoying life. The little man told his story for over an hour. Nothing but misfortune and he didn't complain about anything. Quite the opposite. He even has a sister who fought with another to keep the INSS money he receives because he's invalid... God forbid! I felt so sorry for him that I called Ângelo (the dentist who is the benchmark for prostheses in the Northwest District) to see if he could "pierce" the list of prostheses to make two PPRs for Mr. Falador, but, as I expected, he said he couldn't do it. All the more so because, in this case, the prostheses would have to be made at home, since the patient is unable to travel to Florence (the headquarters of the Specialty Center in the region). I decided to do it myself. Don't they talk about fairness? Well, let social justice be done. I'm going to make the prostheses myself.

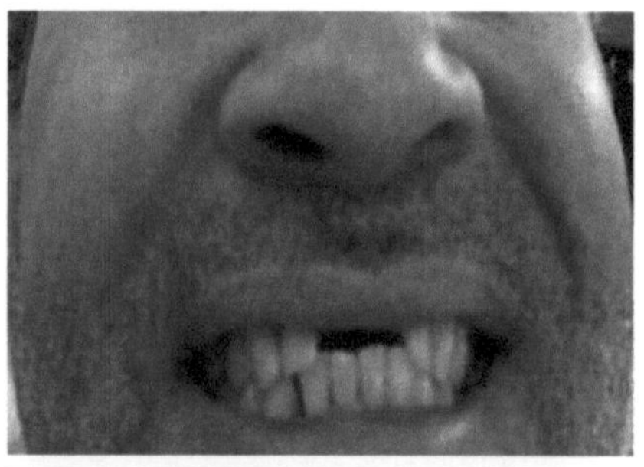

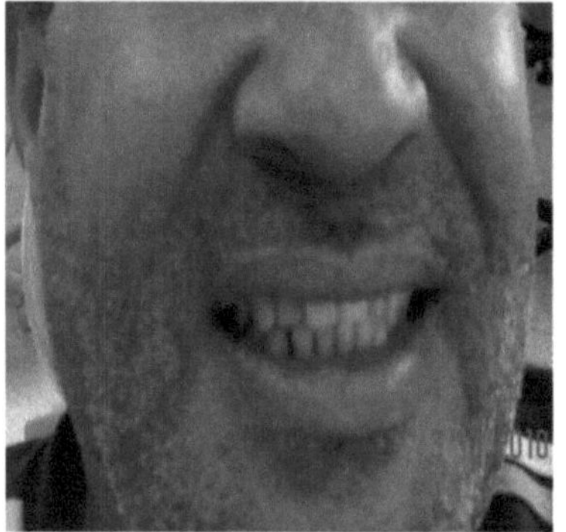

Image 16: "Mr. Talking" had his prosthesis made in a mini-mobile, due to his inability to travel to the Health Center for the various appointments that would be necessary.

16. "Mr. Boiling"

I found this patient in the notebook with the waiting list of patients who want to have prostheses. Mr. A.B., 49, lives in the neighborhood and is a well-known user of the Health Center. The assistants also commented... "Ihhh... are you going to call this guy? He's really angry.... I don't even know why his name is there...". But there aren't many options in the notebook for patients with recent birth dates, so I had no choice, I called!

His wife answered and said she was going to call. I heard her say that it was the "postinho". He quickly answered and asked what it was about. I explained that I was in charge of the prosthesis service and that I was doing some research. I'd like to talk to him and ask him a few questions. The expectation was immediate:

"Are you going to make my bridge?" [referring to the prosthesis].

He said it wasn't his turn yet, but that he'd like to talk. I asked when we could

make an appointment and he said it could be at that moment: "Only if it's now!
"

In less than 10 minutes, he knocked on my door and was very angry. I tried to calm him down and invited him in to sit down. The dentistry room is very large and has four chairs, with no partitions, which takes away the privacy of the users who are there. All the appointments are simultaneous, so sometimes we have 4 users being seen, the 4 dentists who are working, the assistants and often some companions. On this particular day, the room was very full and Mr. A.B. seemed to be on a theater stage ready for a show... He spoke and gesticulated in an agitated and unruly manner. As if he was enjoying having all eyes in the room on him.

He had been without a steady job for a long time, living only from "odd jobs" and had lost his teeth because he didn't have the money to fix them. He had to go to a "perereca ordinària" in the city [referring to the center of Campinas, where there are several popular clinics] because he couldn't go for job interviews without his teeth. Teeth were her calling card. "Without teeth we look sloppy, we look like slobs, thugs, homeless people... How are we going to get an interview without our teeth? Who's going to give me a job like this? [removes prosthesis - "perereca" - and shows mouth without teeth] And then you call at home, but not to say that I'm going to do a decent job, but to ask questions... Do you know what it's like to have no teeth? What it's like to use this thing inside your mouth [shows the "perereca" again]. You can't speak properly, you can't eat... coughing and sneezing, it flies away... you have to hold it... put your hand in front of your mouth so it doesn't fly away... I've had my name on this list for a long time and nothing... I have a 19-year-old son on a bed after he had a motorcycle accident and I ended up being sent away because I only missed work so I could take him to his appointments and exams. How am I supposed to work and leave my wife alone to get him up, change his diaper, clean him and feed him? When I needed them most [referring to the company where I worked] they sent me away without cause... Now I'm unemployed, with no teeth, a paraplegic son, no money... nothing"

In fact, everyone in the room stopped what they were doing and looked at him intently. It was quite an embarrassing situation, but he seemed to be so disgusted that it didn't faze him at all. I tried to calm him down and made him sit down, asked him if he could have a drink and I couldn't hold back a few tears in my eyes. It really was a catastrophic situation...

He also told of the difficulties he had with the town hall to get the help he needed for his son's home visits, the SAD (Sistema de Atendimento Domiciliar) services, the high-cost medicines, in short... there were a lot of problems that ended up breaking him down.

The first thing I managed to say was that he could count on me to make his prosthesis, even if it wasn't his turn. I was going to "beat" the queue... It wouldn't be the first or the last time I'd "break" protocol... He knew that this wouldn't solve his problems in the slightest, but at least it would bring him some comfort...

And so we did.

As the molding and testing sessions went on, we created a closer bond and this made him feel more comfortable telling us about what happened at home, with his son and his family. He ended up agreeing to take part in the research and answered the questions very quickly and succinctly.

His parents had already died and he only had one other sister. The house he lived in belonged to his parents and ended up being his, as his sister got married and moved to São Paulo with her husband. Married for 22 years, he had the son who suffered the motorcycle accident and another 14-year-old girl. He worked as a driver for a construction company, but had been unemployed for over two years. He lived off some "odd jobs" he did, the money he received from the Guarantee Fund ("because the unemployment benefit didn't last long", he said) and truffles that his wife made and sold in the neighborhood.

She said that she had always taken care of her teeth, but after her son's accident she relaxed a lot because she no longer had time for anything. Only to look after her son.

When we finished the prostheses, he was very happy! One less problem, no matter how small and simple it was, seemed like a huge burden to take off his back...

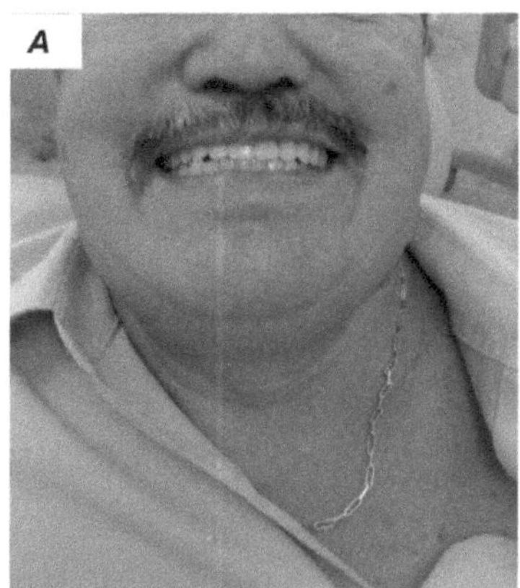

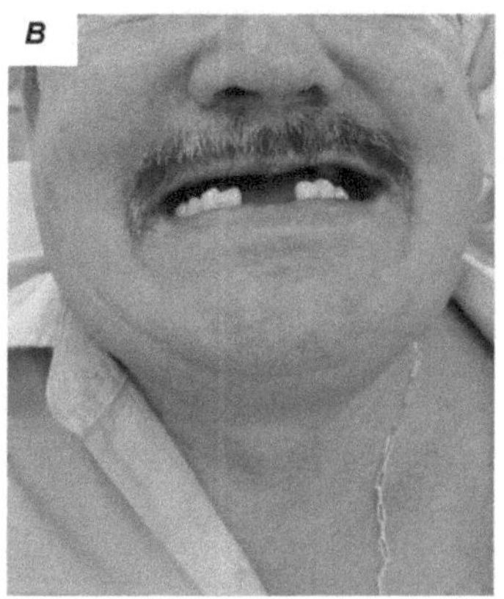

Image 17: "Mr. Boiling" in (A) with the prostheses installed and in (B), before the reception, still on the waiting list. He had a "perereca" which he had made in a folk clinic and would come out while he was talking, eating, coughing, sneezing...

17. *"Sir, not long now"*

A 45-year-old user of the Sao Quirino Health Center, smoker, hypertensive and with great difficulty maintaining good oral hygiene, he was referred to me for removable partial dentures, but with his clinical treatment still incomplete. Dr. "R" wrote a letter explaining this, but at the time I thought it prudent to tell him that his place would be guaranteed, but that he should first complete his treatment at Sao Quirino.

He understood and left...

He returned some time later, with the remaining treatment already completed. On the other hand, a tooth that had already been restored started to hurt. So Dr. "R" thought it best to refer it for endodontic treatment (root canal), but I didn't want to risk starting the impressions, because the tooth in question would be a support for a clip and therefore couldn't be "weakened". Once again, I explained, talked to him and left his place guaranteed until the endodontic treatment was completed. As expected, the tooth was very "fragile" after the treatment and a crown would have to be placed over the tooth to prevent future fracture. The patient couldn't afford this single piece and ended up having a very extensive resurfacing (reconstruction of the element with resin) at the Health Center itself. Between visits, he remained on the waiting list for almost two years. I phoned him to find out if he had completed all the work and, saying yes, he came in for me to examine him. In fact, the restoration had been done, but there was already infiltration and a new cavity was starting in the neck of the same tooth. The difficulty in controlling bacterial plaque, combined with smoking, facilitated this reoccurrence and, for this reason, it has not yet been possible to start prosthetic rehabilitation. We took the opportunity of this last meeting to invite him to take part in the research and he readily accepted.

She told us that she has always taken care of her teeth, but that she started smoking very early, at the age of 14, and that she has a mint habit. "...to get rid of the smell of cigarettes, doctor, I always sucked. Or put something in my mouth. It could be chewing gum, or I could have a coke, anything. I also took a lot of antibiotics as a child. I think this also helped make my teeth weak. Now I'm treating it as Doctor "R" said. I'm really taking care of it.

Soon I'll have to use a license plate.... I don't want to".

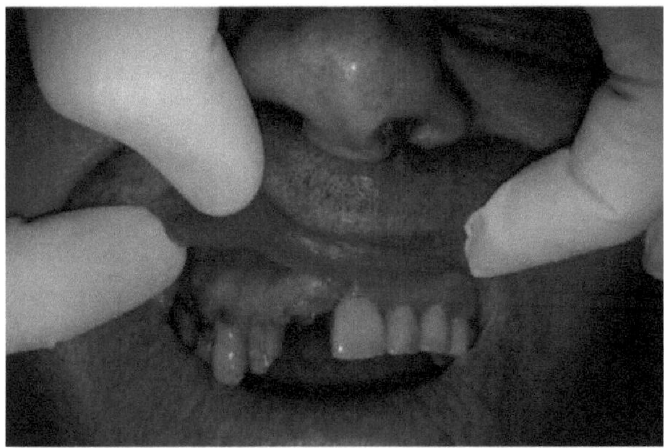

Image 18: "Mr. Falta Pouco" with a previous history of caries, followed by restoration, then endodontics, followed by fracture and, soon, exodontia... Smoking and the difficulty of controlling plaque, coupled with a lack of motivation and adequate guidance to control the disease, led
to tooth loss.

18. "Mr. Died"

We called a user who had been on the waiting list for almost three years and who fit our needs for the table of equivalence between male and female sexes and in the elderly age group. His date of birth was June 7, 1949, and he would have been 68 years old. To our surprise, we received the news that he had died a few months previously.

Another analyzer...

It made us think about this waiting list...

CHAPTER VII: ANALYSIS AND DISCUSSION

According to Mendonça (2001)[106] dental mutilation is considered a relevant health issue, given that it is one of the most prevalent oral diseases and is the result of a past in which dentistry was devoted to relieving pain through extractions and a way of thinking that pointed only to basic care (brushing three times a day and regular visits to the dentist) and sugar reduction/elimination as the "biologicist" ways of solving the problem.

Oral health, however, does not only involve healthy teeth, but much broader issues such as socio-economic and cultural conditions, housing and employment conditions, access to health services, among others. According to Moreira, Nations and Alves (2007, p.1384)[77] "poor people, those with low levels of education and those who are less active in the job market carry dental marks that express an objective reality and a veiled subjective one, whose fundamental aspects have been little studied."

In countries like Brazil, access to dental care is profoundly unequal and there is controversy as to whether investment in specialized services is the solution, according to Chaves et al (2011)[107] , since most of the reduction in health problems would be achieved by improving social indicators, such as schooling, income and occupation, and not necessarily dental care itself.

Since the 1988 Constitution determines that the state is responsible for caring for the health of the population, and the complexity of the health-disease process is added to this, promotion, prevention, diagnosis, treatment and rehabilitation actions should be adequately guaranteed, including tackling access at all levels of care and practicing innovative health attitudes.

However, contrary to expectations, the experience of pain due to tooth loss reveals the difficulty of access to public services, despite the progress represented by the inclusion of oral health in the Family Health Strategy and in the "Smiling Brazil" program of the PNSB.

The study by Cimoes et al (2007)[108] confirms this theory by stating that social class has a significant influence on determining the clinical reasons for tooth loss in the population.

Thus, as a large part of the Brazilian population is living in poverty, it was also expected to find many dental muti- sides, as the possibility of prosthetic replacement is largely limited by economic conditions (Ferreira et al, 2006)[72] .

This situation worsens when associated with the alterations resulting from tooth loss and its repercussions, which should be an object of concern for the professional dental category, according to Silva, Magalhâes and Ferreira (2010, p.814)[76] , but "unfortunately, the approach of professionals, in most cases, only considers the biological and restorative perspectives, that is, the restoration of teeth... neglecting the implications of tooth loss on people's quality of life".

Fonsêca and Junqueira (2014)[9] agree when they state that in dentistry courses, the students' imagination is based on technical centeredness, to the detriment of addressing aspects of the comprehensive health care process.

The individual's mouth and subjectivity are no longer taken into account. "In fact, the toothless person is not considered sick and dental loss is treated differently from the loss of other body structures." (Silva, Magalhaes and Ferreira, 2010 p.816) 6[7]

Silva et al (2010, p.848)[76] agree and state that "the psychological aspects and subjective issues surrounding each situation must be considered as essential as the technical focus."

To this end, welcoming, creating a bond, taking responsibility, promoting a safe diagnosis and interfering in the user's suffering should be therapeutic attitudes. According to Barros and Botazzo (2011, p. 4347)[33] , "in order to understand the other, we need to broaden our professional gaze and listening, which implies adopting new theoretical references and significantly modifying our language and clinical approach.

The struggle to consolidate these concepts must be linked to the construction of innovative health practices, involving management, planning, the work process and a focus on the real needs of users.

When we talk about management and planning, we need to look closely at Institutional Support, which is one of the methodological resources that make up the Paideia Method, Campos (2003)6 and Castro and Campos (2014)[110] , to reformulate the traditional management mechanisms that aim to interfere in the integral formation of subjects, in order to make them rethink and reposition themselves on the levels of emotions and feelings, ideas and knowledge, promoting greater capacity in people to deal with singular issues, which are often unclear, but which emerge as analyzers. As in the case of the child who suffered trauma and lost his permanent front teeth, or in the case of the prosthesis laboratory that remains in another state, kilometers away from the dialogue with the professionals of the prosthesis service in the municipality studied.

Mallmann, Toassi and Abegg (2012)[111] point to the need for an oral health care service, offering dental prostheses, provided by the public sector, with an expanded and organized structure, within the logic and principles that govern the SUS. Otherwise, the pathological stories will continue to bring accounts of the suffering lives of those with mutilated teeth, full of difficulties and pain, as shown in some of the testimonies reported in this work.

To be ready to assist users is to be ready for the encounter (recalling Mendes, Pezzato and Sacardo (2016)[54] , *Every "good encounter" with other bodies, paraphrasing Deleuze in his reading of Spinoza, provokes the generation of power)*, to listen to their stories, to welcome them and, most of the time, to be able to make them feel cared for.

By giving the users a voice, it was as if we had opened windows in a house that had been darkIt was .... as if we had given them a   fresh start... And this was very clear in the stories of the six patients who had already received their prostheses. Their joy and satisfaction at no longer being edentulous is striking, as in the following excerpts:

After I put my teeth in, my husband even kissed me again...

(J.M.B., 25 years old)

When I didn't have my prosthesis, it was difficult even to speak... People stared at us with strange looks on their faces. He pauses and continues: (...). It felt like we were animals... so we spoke like this, you know, with our hands in front of us...

(M.A.R.O., 63 years old)

The best thing about having made the bridge was that the service hired me. Today I'm employed. The manager of (cites the name of a large/known hypermarket) had actually told me that he would only give me a job if I got my teeth fixed.

(R.H.P., 22 years old)

Now you can even eat some ribs, some pork rinds... Too good, right? I know you have to be careful, the doctor explained it to me, but I do eat carefully. Before, it was more like soft food because I had to bite into the gum"

(J.R. 52 years old)

According to Pimenta, L'Abbate and Pezzato (2017, p.55)[112]

The pathographic fragments show that these patients have regained their self-esteem and oral health, by no longer feeling ashamed or embarrassed, by solving relationship and work problems, and by being able to eat properly. This is an effective change in the quality of life of these patients after all the suffering they have endured as a result of the mutilating practices imposed on them throughout their lives and the difficulty of accessing the service.

Recovery through prostheses gave users feelings of achievement, pride, better functionality through their mouths and, of course, their physical appearance ceased to be a stigma (Goffman, 1988)[80]. Tooth loss was perceived as a problem in these people's lives, in other words, it limited chewing, speech, smiling, made it difficult to get a job, as well as feelings of shame and embarrassment, but all these problems seem to have been solved with the prostheses.

Losing teeth is an experience that generates discomfort and limitations, strongly affecting people's lives, but the replacement of lost teeth through prostheses has the potential to add value to the body, restoring balance with the world and making this body, socially marked, accepted. (Bitencourt, Corrêa and Toassi, 2017)[113]

Ferreira et al (2006)[72] also state that the difficulties and limitations imposed on edentulous people can be overcome by placing dental prostheses. These also have the purpose of "replacing part of the body that was once lost". Furthermore, once the abnormality (not having teeth) has been established, it is possible to restore normal mastication by means of a dental prosthesis. It is believed that oral health is also recovered, as individuals can use their mouths again to carry out "social work". (Botazzo, 2006)[114] .

Just like in the case of the "Cashier Girl", who had to wear a prosthesis in order to be accepted as a cashier at the hypermarket. Or "Mrs. Warrior", who told us that she felt like a "bug" and therefore spoke with one hand as if she were covering her mouth. Or like Mrs. "lanky", whose husband no longer wanted to kiss her while she had her teeth out. So, the use of prostheses may not solve the problem of edentulism in our country, but it does make the lack of natural teeth more socially acceptable, as long as it is with the use of prostheses.

According to Bitencourt, Corrêa and Toassi (2017)[113] , stigmatization due to the absence of teeth can affect different areas of people's lives:

... stigmatization comes to have an important influence on the distribution of life opportunities in areas such as income, housing, criminal involvement, health and life. The stigmatized individual becomes aware of how others see him or her, and goes through a process of normalization in order to reduce his or her difference from the prevailing cultural norms. In this way, stigma is linked to the production of social inequalities, since the lack of teeth can lead to the devaluation of certain groups that become socially excluded or devalued in society, making them vulnerable to individual discriminatory experiences based on this stigma. (Bitencourt, Corrêa and Toassi, 2017, the article has already been accepted, but it is not yet published, preventing the pagination)

In the cases of the six patients who were in the process of having their prostheses made, anxiety and expectation were clearly demonstrated, as in the following statements:

My daughter, I'm 82 years old. I've been losing my teeth all my life and I've had to get used to it, like everything else you lose... because I never had the money to go to a private dentist and all they did was pull them out. They could never fix it... I kept losing it until I was like this... Now, I'm going to wait a bit longer for my dentures to arrive, because there's no way, right? You have to make the molds, you have to send them to Curitiba (the city that had an agreement with the prosthesis laboratory accredited by the Campinas municipal government, the site of the research). I understand, you've already explained all this to me... I've waited a long time in this life. Do what, right????

(G.S.A., 82 years old)

This shows the patient's resilience. Bitencourt, Corrêa and Toassi (2017)[113] , state that in old age psychological resources are essential for overcoming adversity in stressful situations. These elements play a central role in protecting the elderly from the influence of loss. "Resilience can be defined as a pattern of adaptive functioning in the face of current and accumulated risks throughout life, which includes biological, socio-economic and psychological risks." These authors conclude by saying that the elderly can change the meaning of the losses and difficulties they have suffered, as well as personal experiences and adverse situations, reducing the level of stressful events, reducing their own negative reactions and maintaining their self-esteem, even when experiencing unfavorable experiences.

(He asked as soon as he heard his name called in the waiting room and his face changed completely when he heard the explanation that he still needed another stage until the prosthesis was completed). I know that the doctor is doing the right thing, but I'd rather come here just once more and take the bridge... Just like in the city [referring to the city center of Campinas, which has several popular clinics]. It's because it's too expensive for me to take three buses to come here all the time...[The region to which he belonged was very far from the place where the prosthesis services are carried out, since this service serves 10 different UBS/regions].

(C.P.N., 58 years old)

There's no way they've replaced my teeth.... What do you mean? If it goes in the box with my name on it, how can it come back changed???? Everything here is difficult... God forbid. Could it be that the men in this laboratory can't even read a name properly? What now? I can't believe it.   Are you sure this mouth

it's not mine? [He asked referring to the prosthesis in the box that had his name labeled on it, but didn't belong to him].

(S.T. 68 years old)

This statement also reveals an analyzer that we have discussed at length. The fact that the municipality chose not to have its own laboratory caused problems for both professionals and users. The deadlines for delivering the work were not always met, there were changes and losses of the boxes containing the prostheses, the distance made dialogue difficult (there are no long-distance telephone calls from the Health Center) and the services often broke down during transportation, which was done inadequately. Thus, according to Lourau (2014)[22] , the structure was revealed ("acting out") as unsatisfactory, although it was maintained by the managers until the end of the contract. It is therefore an analyzer.

However, in the pathographies of the six users who were still waiting on the "waiting lists", the picture was quite different. The speeches echoed pain, sadness and often even revolt. Part of the content of the testimonies that formed the pathographic stories shows the strong impact and negative consequences on the lives of people who have had their teeth mutilated, as can be seen below:

It was taking too long for them to call me to put the bridge in, I thought they weren't even going to call me at home anymore. So I made myself a pererca in town and paid very cheaply...[Patient takes a deep breath and continues] only it's loose... you can't even eat properly or speak... We go to chew it and it stays loose in our mouths. Thank God you called me.

(A.M.S., 43 years old)

According to Silva, Magalhaes and Ferreira (2010)[76], the lack of teeth and the use of inadequate prostheses result in problems with speech, acceptance of physical appearance, with serious repercussions such as lowered self-esteem, difficulties in socializing, a sense of ageing and feelings of humiliation.

I think I'm going to die and they still won't call me. My daughter always goes to the health center to get her blood pressure checked and she always asks the dentist if it's my turn, but they always say it's going to take a while because there's only one dentist to make the dentures for a lot of people.

(C.P.S., 58 years old)

In this speech, the patient also referred to the fact that the municipality has only one dental surgeon to make prostheses for each of the 5 regions of the city, and that there are around 10 UBSs in each of the regions.

Not having teeth is bad, but what's worse is knowing that you don't have them because of the theft... There's money, right? But they steal it all and then there's no money left for health. They'd rather steal the taxes we pay than hire more people to make dentures for us... (J.S. 72 years old)

Again we quote Ferreira et a (2006, p.211)[72] :

If, on the one hand, the Experience of Pain indicates restricted access to dental services, on the other, Tooth Loss denounces the existence of a mutilating practice imposed by public health services to solve the pain. This category also includes dental prostheses, the possibility of which is limited by economic conditions.

We agree with Santos and Assis (2006)[115] that the practice of oral health is full of conflicts and contradictions, as well as being an unfinished process under construction, but we have to take into account the unique aspects of individuals facing the challenges of the health/disease process so that these limits of oral health practices can be overcome.

CHAPTER VIII: FINAL CONSIDERATIONS

The framework of Institutional Analysis in Public Health has been used more consistently in Brazil since the 2000s, especially in disciplines such as Planning and Management in Health Services and Social Sciences in Health. In 2002, L'Abbate introduced the IA discipline in the Post-Graduate Program in Collective Health at the DSC/FCM/Unicamp and created a research group with the CNPq, a Research Directory, entitled "Institutional Analysis & Collective Health", which has greatly contributed to demonstrating the potential of this reference, which can be seen in the Institutional Analysis & Collective Health Collection published in 2013, referred to in this work.

The Oral Health Policy of the Campinas Municipal Health Department is an institution that is "materialized" in the Prosthesis Service, so we analyzed its social and organizational reality. To do this, we used the concepts of Analyzer and Implication, mainly in the context of AI.

My implications were highlighted in the first chapter of this thesis and I tried to make the diaries visible as a way of articulating my individual dimensions with the organizational and institutional interfaces of the service. The analyzers were seen throughout the thesis and revealed the "carelessness" of the Health Department, showing that what seemed to be organized, in fact, is not. The broader analyses were built up as the pathographies took shape and narrower questions arose.

Throughout the research, I was able to identify the need to go far beyond the policies already in place, so that it would be possible for professionals in the Prosthesis Service to interfere positively and responsibly in the suffering of the people who depend on the service.

As stated by Pimenta, L'Abbate and Pezzato (2017, p.58)[112] , "(...) it is imperative to reorganize the Municipal Oral Health Policy of Campinas in order to place the user at the center of the production of care, in order to meet their needs, since the results point to the insufficiency and inadequacy of the existing service."

Regarding aspects of the oral health of mutilated tooth users who had used, were using or were waiting to use the Prosthesis Service of the Eastern District of the municipality of Campinas, it was concluded that those who had already had their prostheses fitted had had their oral health restored; those who were in the process of having their prostheses made were still uncomfortable and anxious to be able to restore their oral health as soon as possible by installing the new prostheses; and finally, those who remained on the waiting list were dissatisfied, with difficulties in speaking, eating and relationships due to their aesthetics. They had a diminished quality of life, low self-esteem and were often disgusted with politics and the politicians in power.

The work process of the Prosthesis Service, within the context of a Basic Health Unit, has favorable implications for the access of many patients, as in the case of the "Man from the Ombudsman's Office" who was referred to us directly by the psychiatrist from the Health Center, or the "Mrs. Polyoxy", who was always at the Unit at the request of the coordinator, or the "Mrs. Warrior" who ended up meeting another user who had just been seen. Mrs. Warrior" who was always in the Unit to have her blood pressure checked and ended up meeting another user who had just been seen at the prosthesis service, which she didn't even know existed... This led to the possibility of putting her name on the waiting list.

The potential of the "SUS Campinas Prosthesis Service" is enormous, because oral health needs are expressed very intensely in population groups linked to the lower social classes. From the patient's point of view, untreated tooth decay, severe pain, infections and suffering result in tooth extractions throughout the individual's life, and the possibility of rehabilitation is the only way to restore lost adversity and ambiguity.

Finally, with a view to instituting ways of qualifying the service so that it is more resolutive and effective, we can list a few possibilities:

1. Guarantee an oral health professional in each of the Basic Health Units to make prostheses for the mutilated teeth in the region, as recommended by the PNSB, including during vacations and/or leaves of absence of the appointed

dentist.

2. If the measure proposed in the previous item is not possible, increase the training of dental surgeons in each Basic Health Unit to solve problems related to the adjustment and adaptation of new or old prostheses, reducing the flow of patients in the reference professional's agenda.

3. Effectively carry out strategic planning and management so that there is no shortage of essential supplies for the service or purchases of inappropriate materials.

4. Increasing regular dialogue and exchange of knowledge with management, so that specific problems can be solved before they become challenges to a hegemonic model that is maintained in a naturalized way.

5. Provide conditions for reception and triage to be equitable for users on waiting lists, so that patients in only adequate conditions and within the protocol are referred for referral. Unique cases should be treated with greater care and attention.

6. Ensure the installation of an in-house laboratory, as envisioned by the PNSB, with a prosthetist hired by the municipality, to allow for adequate technical work and logistics for getting prostheses to and from their laboratory phases/stages.

7. If it is not possible to carry out the proposal in the previous item, a laboratory of technical excellence should be hired, in reasonable proximity to the locations of the Prosthetic Services.

8. Ensure that each UBS hires a professional oral health technician or assistant to perform their skills and functions, in order to optimize the time/quality of the dental professional.

These possibilities for qualifying the SUS Campinas prosthesis service could undoubtedly ensure "No smile less" (Radis, 2017)[116] , according to the cover story in this issue of the magazine, because oral health is capable of guaranteeing citizenship and quality of life to those who are socially excluded due to dental mutilation.

BIBLIOGRAPHICAL REFERENCES

1.   Oliveira, MAC, Egry, EY. The Historicity of Interpretative Theories of the Health-Disease Process. Rev Esc Enf USP. mar 2000; v.34, n.1:9-15.

2.   Giudice ACMP. Popular participation in health services: a way to increase access and adherence to treatment. Dissertation (Master's Degree). State University of Campinas, 2008; Piracicaba School of Dentistry.

3.   Fadel CB, Saliba NA. Social representations as an information tool for collective oral health. RGO - Rev. Gaûcha Odontologia. Oct/Dec.2010; Porto Alegre, v.58, n.4: 521-526.

4.   Narvai PC, Frazâo P. Oral Health Policies in Brazil. In: Moysés ST, Kriger L, Moysés SJ. Family oral health: working with evidence. Ed. Artes Médicas. 2008; 308p.

5.   Foucault M. O nascimento da clinica. (Traduçâo de Roberto Machado) 5ed. Rio de Janeiro: Editora Forense Universitària.

6.   Campos GWS (org). Health Paideia. Sao Paulo: Editora Hucitec, 2003.

7.   L'Abbate S, Mourao LC, Pezzato LM (org). Institutional Analysis and Collective Health. Sao Paulo: Hucitec, 2013.

8.   Donnangelo MCFA. Research in Collective Health in Brazil - the 70s. In: Teaching Public Health, Preventive and Social Medicine in Brazil. Rio de Janeiro: ABRASCO, 1983. Notebook 2: 17-35.

9.   Fonsêca GS Junqueira SR. Work Education for Health Program. Curitiba/PR: Editora Appris, 2014, 245p.

10. Calado GS. The inclusion of the oral health team in the family health program: main advances and challenges. [Master's dissertation]. Rio de Janeiro: National School of Public Health, Oswaldo Cruz Foundation; 2002.

11. Brazil, Ministry of Health. Health Care Secretariat. Department of Primary Care. National primary care policy / Ministry of Health, Department of Health Care,

Department of Health Care. - Brasilia: Ministry of Health, 2006.

1.1. Ministry of Health. Health Care Secretariat. Department of Primary Care. Coordination of Monitoring and Evaluation of Primary Care, Brasilia: Ministry of Health 2004.

1.2. Ministry of Health. Portaria MS/GM n.1444, de 28 de dezembro de 2000. Diàrio Oficial da Uniâo, Brasilia/DF, dec.2000, n.250E, Sec. 1, p.85.

14. Frazâo P, Narvai PC. Twenty years of the Unified Health System: advances and challenges for oral health. Cad. Saùde Pùblica. 2009 Apr; vol.25: no.4: 712-714.

15. . Oral health in the Unified Health System: 20 years of struggle for a public policy. Saùde em Debate. 2009 Jan/Apr; vol 33: no. 81: 64-71.

16. Baldani MH, Fadel C, Possamai T, Queiroz MGS. The inclusion of dentistry in the Family Health Program in the State of Paranà, Brazil. Cad. Saùde Pùblica. Jul-Aug, 2005; 21 (4): 10261035.

17. Ferraz GA, Leite ICG. Home Visit Instruments: Dentistry's Approach to the Family Health Strategy. Rev. APS. Apr/Jun 2016; 19(2): 302-314.

18. Viana IB, Martelli PJ, Pimentel C. Analysis of the Evolution of Oral Health Teams in the Family Health Strategy in Pernambuco from 2001 to 2009. In J Dent. 2011 Oct/Dec; 10(4): 242-248

19. Lourau R. The instituting against the instituted. In: Altoé S. (org). René Lourau: Full-time Institutional Analyst. Hucitec. 2004; 283p.

20. Guillier Samson D. Implication: des discours d'hier aux pratiques d'aujourd'hui. Les Cahiers de l'implication. Revue d'analyse institutionnelle. 1997; no 1: 17-29.

21. Monceau G. Implication, overimplication and professional implication. Fractal, Revista de Psicologia. jan/jun 2008; v.20, no1: 19-26.

22. Lourau R. Institutional analysis. [Translation by Mariano Ferreira]. 3 ed. Vozes, 2014

23. Lapassade G, Lourau R. Keys to Sociology. Ed. Civilizaçâo Brasileira, 1972.

24. Coimbra CMB, Nascimento ML. Analysis of Implications: challenging our practices of knowledge/power. In: Geisler ARR, Abraâo LA, Coimbra CMB (eds). Subjectivities, violence and human rights: producing new devices in health. Ed UFF. 2008; 143-153.

25. Barbier R. Action research in the educational institution. Zahar. 1985.

26. Monceau G. Analyzing its implications in the scientific institution: an alternative path. Estudos e Pesquisas em Psicologia. 2010; 10 (1): 13-30, Accessed at: http://www.revispsi.uerj.br

27. Romagnoli RC. The concept of implication and institutionalist intervention research. Psicologia & Sociedade. 2014; 26 (1): 44-52.

28. Botazzo C. Innovation in the Production of Oral Health Care. Possibilities for a new approach in the dental clinic for the Unified Health System. [Research project] approved under MCTI/CNPq/MS-SCTIE-Decit call number 10/2012.

29. Campos GWS. A method for the analysis and co-management of collectives. Sâo Paulo: Editora Hucitec. 2000.

30. Starfield B. Primary Care: balancing health needs, services and technology. Brasilia, 2002. UNESCO, Ministry of Health.

31. Kovaleski DF, Freitas SFT, Botazzo C. Disciplinarization of the mouth, the autonomy of the individual in the society of work. Ciência & Saùde Coletiva. 2006; 11(1): 97-103

32. Campos RO. Qualitative Research in Collective Health Policies, Planning and Management. In: Barros NF, Cecatti JG, Turato ER. Qualitative Research in Health - Multiple Views. (org) Campinas: Unicamp. 2005

33. Barros RS, Botazzo C. Subjectivities and the clinic in primary care. Narratives, life stories and social reality. Ciência & Saùde Coletiva. 2011;16(11): 4337-4348

34. Sciliar M. History of the concept of health. Physis [online]. 2007;   v.17, n.1: 29-41 Available at http://dx.doi.org/10.1590/S0103-73312007000100003

35. Luz MT. Complexity of the Collective Health field: multidisciplinarity, interdisciplinarity, and transdisciplinarity of knowledge and practices - socio-historical analysis of a paradigmatic trajectory. Health and Society. Apr/Jun 2009; v18, no 2

36. Merhy, EE, Feuerwerker LCM. A new look at health technologies: a contemporary need. In : Mandarino ACS, Gomberg E, (org). New technologies and health. Sâo Cristóvào: Editora UFS. 2009; 29-56

37. Allison PJ, Lovker D, Feine JS. Quality of life: a dynamic construct. Soc. Sci. Med. 1997; 45: 221-230.

38. Bendo CB, Martins CC, Pordeus IA, Paiva SM. Impact of oral conditions on the quality of life of individuals. Revista Assoc. Paul. Cir. Dent. 2014; 68 (3): 189-193.

39. Guattari F. Chaosmosis: A New Aesthetic Paradigm. Editora 34 Ltda. Sâo Paulo, 1992. (Translated by Ana Lùcia Oliveira and Lùcia Clàudia Leâo)

40. Simonetti A. Beyond Sadness. Secrets of the Mind magazine. 2016.

41. Lawrence HP, Thomson MW, Broadbent J M, Poulton R. Oral health-related quality of life in a birth cohort of 32 years old. Community Dent Oral Epidemiol. 2008; 36: 305-316.

42. Traverso-Yépez M, Morais NA. Claiming the subjectivity of users of the Primary Health Care Network: towards a humanization of care. Cad. Saùde Pùblica. jan-feb, 2004; 20 (1): 8088.

43. Souza ECF. Training and Work in Dentistry: Expanding the Clinic to Build a New Culture of Oral Health Care. Text presented at the III State Oral Health Conference, in the thematic panel "Training and Work in Oral Health". Natal/RN, May 28, 2004

44. Souza ECF. Mouths, cancer and subjectivities - Pathographies under analysis. [PhD thesis in Collective Health]. Faculty of Medical Sciences, UNICAMP/SP, 2003.

45. Franco TB, Merhy EE. Work, production of care and subjectivity in health. Sâo Paulo: Editora Hucitec. 2013.

46.   Deleuze G, Guattari F. On Anti-Oedipus. J. Psychiatry. 1972

47.   Merhy EE. In search of tools to analyze Health Technologies: information and the day-to-day life of a service, questioning and managing health work. In: Merhy EE, Onoko R. (org). Acting in Health: a challenge for the public. 2nd ed. Sâo Paulo: Editora Hucitec. 2002.

48.   Botazzo C. Da Arte Dentària. São Paulo: Editora Hucitec, 2000.

49.   . Oral health in the context of the Family Health Strategy: helping to promote health for individuals, groups and families. In: Moysés ST, Kriger L, Moysés SJ. (org). Family oral health: working with evidence. Sâo Paulo: Ed. Artes Médicas, 2008.

50.   . Bucalidade. Pro-Odonto Prevençâo. 2013; 6(4): 9-55

51.   . Subjectivity and Dental Practice. Theoretical and political notes. Workshop at the XII Paulista Congress of Public Health. October 22-26, 2011.

52.   Kovaleski DF. The Disciplinarization of the Mouth: from the technologies of the "self" to the regime of life. [Master's dissertation] - Federal University of Santa Catarina, Health Sciences Center, 2004.

53.   Martines WRV, Machado AL. Producing care and subjectivity. Rev Brasileira de Enfermagem. Mar/Apr 2010; 63(2): 328-333.

54.   Mendes R, Pezzato LM, Sacardo DP. Research-intervention in health promotion; methodological challenges of researching "with". Ciência & Saùde Coletiva. 2016; 21(6): 1737-1745.

55.   Botazzo C. Innovation in the Production of Oral Health Care. Possibilities for a new approach in the dental clinic for the Unified Health System. Technical Report. University of Sao Paulo. Call MCTI/CNPq/MS- SCTIE-DECID no 10/2012

56.   Merhy EE. In search of quality in health services: open-door health services and the technical-care model in defense of life. Health in Debate. 1994; 76 (3): 117-160.

57.   Merhy EE. In search of quality in health services: open-door health

services and the technical-care model in defense of life. In: Cecilio LC. Inventing Change in Health. Sao Paulo: Editora Hucitec, 1997; 117-160.

58. Mendes R. Healthy Cities in Brazil and Participatory Processes: The Cases of Jundiai and Maceió [PhD thesis] Faculdade de Saùde Pùblica da Universidade de Sao Paulo.1999.

59. Ministry of Health. SB Brasil Project 2010: oral health conditions of the Brazilian population - main results. Brasilia: Ministry of Health; 2011.

60. Lewandowski A,Bós AJG. Oral health status and the need for dental prostheses in the long-lived elderly. Rev. Assoc. Paul Cir. Dent. 2014; 68(2): 155-158.61

61. Brazil, Ministry of Health. National Oral Health Division. Epidemiological survey on oral health-Brazil, urban area, 1986. Brasilia: Ministry of Health, 1988.

62. Pinto VG. Epidemiology of Oral Diseases in Brazil. In: Krieger L. (org) Promoçao da Saùde Bucal. Sao Paulo: Editora Artes Médicas, 1988; 27-42.

63. Morita MC, Haddad AE, Araujo ME. Current Profile and Trends of Brazilian Dental Surgeons. Maringà: Ed Dental Press; 2016.

64. L'Abbate S. Institutional Analysis and Intervention: a brief reference to the social and historical genesis of an articulation and its application in Collective Health. Mnemosine. 2012; v.8 n.1: 194219.

65. The money analyzer in group work at a University Hospital in Campinas, São Paulo: revealing and unveiling institutional contradictions. In: Rodrigues HBC, Altoé S. (org). Saùde e Loucura n° 8. Anâlise Institucional, Sâo Paulo: Editora Hucitec. 2004; 79-99.

66. Dobies DV, L'Abbate S. Resistance as an analyzer of mental health in Campinas (SP): contributions from Institutional Analysis. Health in Debate. July/September 2016; v.40, no. 110: 120-133.

67. Lapassade G. El analizador y el analista. Barcelona Gedisa S.A. 1979.

68. Hess R, Savoye A. L'Analyse Institutionnelle, (Que sais-je?). 2 ed, Paris,

PUF. 1993; ch. IX: 97-111. (Translated by Ana Lùcia Abrahâo da Silva and Lùcia Cardoso Mourâo. Proofreading by Solange L'Abbate)

69. Sheiham A, Moysés S J. The role of oral health professionals in Health Promotion. In: Buischi Y P. Promoçâo de saúde bucal na clinica odontológica. Sâo Paulo: Editora Artes Médicas, 2000.

70. Aerts D, Abegg C, Cesa K. The role of the dental surgeon in the Unified Health System. Ciência & Saùde coletiva. 2004; 9(1): 131 - 138.

71. Almeida AB, Alves MS, Leite IC. Reflections on the challenges of dentistry in the Unified Health System. Rev. Atençâo Prim. Saùde. 2010; v 13, no 1: 126-132.

72. Ferreira AAA, Piuvezam G, Werner CWA, Alves MSCF. Pain and tooth loss: social representations of oral health care. Ciência & Saùde Coletiva. 2006; 11 (1): 211-218.

73. Martino LVS. The National Oral Health Policy in municipalities in the Metropolitan Region of São Paulo in the first decade of the 21st century. [Master's dissertation in Public Health]. School of Public Health, University of São Paulo/SP, 2011.

74. Araùjo ME, Zilbovicius C. Health work: looking at and experiencing the SUS in everyday life. *Trab. educ. saùde*. Sep 2004; vol.2 no.2: 388-391.

75. Guimaraes MM, Marcos B. Expectation of tooth loss in different social classes. Revista do Conselho Regional de Odontologia de Minas Gerais. 1996; 2(1):16-20.

76. Silva MES, Magalhaes CS, Ferreira EF. Tooth Loss and the Expectation of Prosthetic Replacement: a qualitative study. Ciência & Saùde coletiva. 2010; 15 (3): 813-820.

77. Moreira TP, Nations MK, Alves MSCF. Teeth of Inequality: marks of the lived experience of poverty in the community of Dendê, Fortaleza, Cearà, Brazil. Cad. Saùde Pùblica. jun, 2007; 23(6): 1383-1392.

78. Souza ECF. Illness, Narrative, Subjectivities. Pathographies as a Tool for the Clinic. Editora da UFRN, 2011.

79. Vargas AMD, Paixao HH. Tooth loss and its significance in the quality of life of adult users of public oral health services at the Boa Vista Health Center in Belo Horizonte. Ciência & Saùde Coletiva. 2005; 10(4): 1015-1024.

80. Goffman E. Stigma: notes on the manipulation of damaged identity. Editora Guanabara Koogan. Rio de Janeiro, 1988.

81. Journal of the Federal Council of Dentistry: Apr-May-Jun 2012; n° 103

82. Folha de Sâo Paulo newspaper. 01/07/2015. http://acervo.folha.uol.com.br/fsp/2015/07/01/21/ accessed on 10/10/2017.

83. http://www.saude.campinas.sp.gov.br/saude (accessed September 2017)

84. L'Abbate S. Right to Health. Discourses and Practices in the Construction of the SUS. Sâo Paulo: Editora Hucitec, 2010.

85. Manfredini MA. Oral Health in the Family Health Strategy in Campinas, SP. In: Moysés ST, Kriger L, Moysés SJ. Family oral health: working with evidence. Ed. Artes Médicas, 2008.

86. Stake RE. Qualitative Research - studying how things work. Artmed Editora S.A., 2011.

87. Pinheiro R, Guizard FL, Machado FRS, Gomes RS. Health Demand and Right to Health: Freedom or Necessity? Some Considerations on the Constituent Links of Integrality Practices. In Pinheiro R, Mattos RA. Construçâo Social da Demanda, 2 Ed., Rio de Janeiro: CEPESC/UERJ: ABRASCO, 2010.

88. Cecilio LCO. Health Needs as a Structuring Concept in the Struggle for Comprehensiveness and Equity in Care In: Pinheiro R, Roseni, Mattos, Ruben Araùjo. The meanings of comprehensiveness in health care. Rio de Janeiro, IMS ABRASCO, 2001.

89. Minayo MCS. The challenge of knowledge: qualitative research in health. 14 ed. Sâo Paulo: Editora Hucitec, 2014.

90. Pope C, Mays N. Pesquisa Qualitativa na Atençâo à Saù, 2 ed.

91. Barros NF, Cecatti JG, Turato ER. (org): Pesquisa Qualitativa em Saùde

Mùltiplos Olhares. Faculdade de Ciências Médicas/Unicamp, Editora Komedi, 2005.

92. L'Abbate S. Institutional Analysis and Health Education: a productive dialog. Boletim do Instituto de Saúde n. dedicated to Health Education. SES/SP, 1997.

93. Pezzato LM, L'Abbate S. The use of diaries as an intervention tool of Institutional Analysis: enhancing reflections in the daily routine of Collective Oral Health. Physis Rev. Saùde Coletiva. 2011;21(4): 1297 -1314.

94. Mendes R, Pezzato LM, Sacardo DP. Intervention research in health promotion: methodological challenges of researching "with". Ciência & saùde Coletiva. 2016; 21(6): 1737-1745.

95. Passos E, Barros RBA. The Construction of the Clinical Plan and the Concept of Transdisciplinarity. Psicologia: Teoria e Pesquisa. 2000; v.16, n.1: 71-79.

96. Barbier R. Action Research. Brasilia: Plano Editora, 2002.

97. Pezzato LM, L'Abbate S. An action-intervention research in Collective Oral Health: contributing to the production of new analyses. Health and Society. Jun 2012; vol.21, no.2: 686-398.

98. Childs V, Franklin F, Kemp P. Action research in social services and health care settings. Cambridge. Anglia Polytechnic University, 1997.

99. Rocha ML, Aguiar KF. Research-intervention and the production of new analyses Psicologia: ciência e profissâo [on line]. 2003; v.23, n.4: 64-73.

100. Haguette TMF. Qualitative methodologies in sociology. 14 ed. Petrópolis. Vozes, 2013.

101. Castiel LD. The hole and the ostrich: the singularity of human illness. Campinas, SP. Papirus, 1994

102. Entralgo PL. Clinical history. History and theory of pathographic reporting. Madrid. Editoria Triacastela, 1998.

103. Kovaleski DF, Freitas SFT. Pathographic stories as a form of field

research report. Saùde &Transformaçâo Social / Health & Social Change. Federal University of Santa Catarina. 2010; vol. 1, n. 1: 61-69.

104. Pezzato LM, Prado GVT. Research-Action and Research-Intervention: Approaches, Distances, Conjugations. In.

L'Abbate S, Mourao LC, Pezzato LM. (org). Institutional Analysis and Collective Health. Hucitec Editora. Sâo Paulo, 2013.

105. Jornal da Associaçâo Paulista de Cirurgioes Dentistas (APCD Jornal - February 2016)

106. Mendonça TC. Tooth mutilation: rural workers' conceptions of responsibility for tooth loss. Cad. Saùde Pùblica. Rio de Janeiro, Nov-Dec, 2001; 17(6):1545-1547.

107. Chavês SC, Cruz DN, Barros SG, Figueiredo AL. Evaluation of the supply and use of dental specialties in public secondary care services in Bahia, Brazil. Cad. Saùde Pùblica. jan/2011; 27(1): 143-154.

108. Cimoes R, Jûnior AFC, Souza EHA, Gusmâo ES. Influence of social class on the clinical reasons for tooth loss. Ciência & Saùde Coletiva. 2007; 12(6): 1691-1696.

109. Silva MES, Villaça EL, Magalhaes CS, Ferreira EF. Impact of tooth loss on quality of life. Ciência & Saùde Coletiva. 2010; 15(3): 841-850.

110. Castro CP, Campos GWS. Paideia Institutional Support as a strategy for permanent health education. Trab.educ.saùde. 2014; v12, no 1: 29-50

111. Mallmann FH, Toassi RF, Abegg C. Epidemiological profile of the use and need for dental prostheses in individuals aged 50-74 years, living in three "Health Districts" of Porto Alegre, State of Rio Grande do Sul, Brazil, in 2008. Epidemiol. Serv. Saùde. 2012; v 21, no 1: 1-11.

112. Pimenta ACM, L'Abbate S, Pezzato LM. Pathographic histories of dental mutilations in a prosthesis service of the Unified Health System. Rev. Ciênc. Méd. Campinas, May/Aug 2017; 26(2): 49-59.

113. Bitencourt FV, Toassi RFC, Corrêa HW. Experiences of tooth loss in adult

and elderly users of primary health care. Cien.Saùde Colet [periodical on the internet] (2017/ Jul).[Cited on 26/10/2017]. Available from: www.cienciaesaudecoletiva.com.br/artigos/experiencias-de- dental-loss-in-adult-and-elderly-users-of-primary-health-care/16295

114. Botazzo C. On oral health: notes for research and contribution to the debate. Ciência & Saùde Coletiva. 2006: v 11(1): 7-17.

115. Santos AM, Assis MMA. From fragmentation to integrality: building and (un)building oral health practice in the Family Health Program (PSF) of Alagoinha, BA. Ciência & Saùde Coletiva. 2006; 11(1): 53-61.

116. Nothing Pays for a Smile. Radis - Fiocruz. Nov/2017; 16-22.

ANNEXES: INFORMED CONSENT FORM

Project title: The Institutionalization of the Prosthesis Service in Campinas/SP and the Subjectivity of Mutilated Dentists.

Principal Investigator: Ana Claudia Moutella Pimenta Giudice

Institution: State University of Campinas/Unicamp

Contact numbers: (19) 2121-4667 and (19) 99116-0033

Contact e-mail: anacmpg@yahoo.com.br and anacmpg1@gmail.com

Name of volunteer

R.G.:

Date of birth:

You are being invited to take part in the research project entitled "The Institutionalization of the Prosthesis Service in Campinas/SP and the Subjectivity of Mutilated Dentists", under the responsibility of researcher Ana Claudia Moutella Pimenta Giudice, under the supervision of Professor Solange L'Abbate, whose main objective is to investigate the process of institutionalization of the prosthesis service in the municipality of Campinas/SP, considering policies, the structure of services, as well as practices and assistance in the face of oral health needs from the subject-patient point of view.

We need your agreement, informing you that at any time, for any reason, explained or not, you can give up, leave/withdraw from the research without any burden or damage to you. We also inform you that the recorded statements and images will not be identified by name under any circumstances and will only be used for scientific purposes such as publication or presentation at events.

I declare that I have been informed of the motives and objectives of the research and that my anonymity has been guaranteed, as well as the right to not participate or to withdraw at any stage of the development of this project, without this causing me any harm. I also declare that I have agreed spontaneously.

Researcher's responsibility:

I assure you that I have complied with the requirements of Resolution 466/2012 CNS/MS and complementary resolutions in drawing up the protocol and obtaining this Informed Consent Form. I also assure that I have explained and provided a copy of this document to the participant. I inform you that the study was approved by the REC to which the project was submitted. I undertake to use the material and data obtained in this research exclusively for the purposes set out in this document or in accordance with the consent given by the participant.

(Signature of Researcher)

If you have any complaints about your participation in the study, you can contact the secretary of the Research Ethics Committee (CEP): Rua Tessàlia Vieira de Camargo, 126; CEP: 13083-887 Campinas/SP, telephone (19) 3521-8936; email:

cep@fcm.unicamp.br

Campinas, / /

(Signature of the Volunteer - if under 18, the signature and ID of the parent/legal guardian is required)

Authorization document for the survey at Campinas City Hall

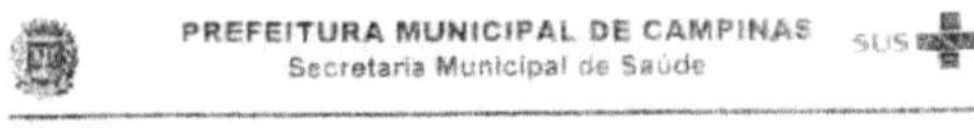

AUTORIZAÇÃO

Autorizo a realização da pesquisa de doutorado intitulada "**A Institucionalização do Serviço de Prótese de Campinas/SP e a Subjetividade dos Mutilados Dentais**" que tem por objetivo investigar o processo de institucionalização do serviço de prótese no município de Campinas/SP, considerando as políticas, a estruturação dos serviços, além das práticas e da assistência em face das necessidades de saúde bucal do ponto de vista do sujeito – paciente.

Declaro estar ciente que esta pesquisa será realizada no Centro de Saúde Costa e Silva – Distrito Leste pela pesquisadora Ana Claudia Moutella Pimenta Giudice sob a orientação da Profa. Dr. Solange L'Abbate.

Declaro ainda que esta pesquisa teve início após um estudo multicêntrico denominado "Inovação na Produção do Cuidado em Saúde Bucal: possibilidades de uma nova abordagem na clínica odontológica para o Sistema Único de Saúde" que foi aprovada pelo Comitê de Ética e Pesquisa da Faculdade de Odontologia de São Paulo/Plataforma Brasil número do parecer 501069.

Campinas, 03 de outubro de 2013

Carmino Antonio de Souza
Secretário Municipal de Saúde

Research Ethics Committee Approval Document

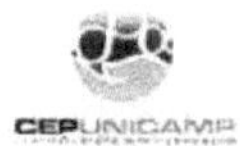

COMITÊ DE ÉTICA EM
PESQUISA DA UNICAMP -
CAMPUS CAMPINAS

PARECER CONSUBSTANCIADO DO CEP

DADOS DO PROJETO DE PESQUISA

Título da Pesquisa: A Institucionalização do Serviço de Prótese de Campinas/SP e a Subjetividade dos Mutilados Dentais

Pesquisador: Ana Cláudia Moutella Pimenta Giudice

Área Temática:

Versão: 4

CAAE: 54809916.8.0000.5404

Instituição Proponente: Faculdade de Ciências Medicas - UNICAMP

Patrocinador Principal: Financiamento Próprio

DADOS DO PARECER

Número do Parecer: 1.668.950

Apresentação do Projeto:

Segundo informa a equipe de pesquisa: "Este projeto de doutorado tem como objetivo analisar o processo de institucionalização do serviço de prótese dental, no municipio de Campinas/SP, considerando as políticas, a estruturação dos serviços, além das práticas e da assistência em face das necessidades de saúde bucal do ponto de vista do sujeito paciente. O percurso metodológico será a Análise Institucional, com a utilização de diários realizados pela pesquisadora e entrevistas com os usuários mutilados dentais do SUS da região Leste do município em questão, a fim de se construir as histórias patográficas dos mesmos. O conceito de patografia desenvolvido por Anne Hawkins, 1998, trata de estudar os modos como os individuos acometidos por afecções graves, procuram ordenar os eventos produzindo narrativas em que se estabelecem atribuições causais, motivações e papéis aos agentes. Segundo L`Abbate 2012, a Análise Institucional tem por objetivo compreender uma determinada realidade social, organizacional, a partir dos discursos e práticas dos sujeitos. Espera-se então, através das patografias e da análise institucional identificar as dimensões subjetivas dos pacientes mutilados dentais que utilizaram/utilizam o serviço, compreendendo o processo de trabalho dentro do contexto vigente, analisando as potencialidades e dificuldades na ótica dos sujeitos-pacientes, apontando possibilidades instituintes de qualificação."

Endereço: Rua Tessália Vieira de Camargo, 126
Bairro: Barão Geraldo   **CEP:** 13.083-887
UF: SP   **Município:** CAMPINAS
Telefone: (19)3521-8936   **Fax:** (19)3521-7187   **E-mail:** cep@fcm.unicamp.br

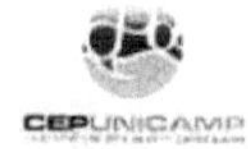 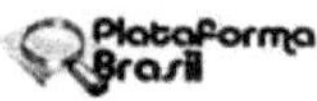

Objetivo da Pesquisa:

Objetivo Primário:

Investigar o processo de institucionalização do serviço de prótese, no município de Campinas/SP, considerando as políticas, a estruturação dos serviços, além das práticas e da assistência em face das necessidades de saúde bucal do ponto de vista sujeito-paciente

Objetivo Secundário:

A) Identificar as dimensões subjetivas dos pacientes mutilados dentais que se utilizaram/utilizam do Serviço de Prótese do SUS Campinas.

B)Compreender o processo de trabalho do Serviço de Prótese instituído na Secretaria da Saúde, dentro do contexto vivente.

C) Analisar a potencialidade da instituição "Serviço de Prótese do SUS Campinas" em usuários mutilados dentais, na ótica do sujeito/paciente.

D) Apontar possibilidades instituintes de qualificação no Serviço de Prótese.

Avaliação dos Riscos e Benefícios:

Segundo informações da pesquisadora:

Riscos:

Não há riscos previsíveis

Benefícios:

Não há benefícios diretos a pessoa, mas espera-se que a pesquisa possa fornecer dados para qualificação do serviço e aumentar o acesso para outros usuários.

Comentários e Considerações sobre a Pesquisa:

Informa a equipe de pesquisa sobre a metodologia: "A pesquisa será realizada a partir de entrevistas com usuários do Sistema Único de Saúde (SUS) que utilizam, utilizaram e estão na "lista de espera" do Serviço de Prótese Dental do Distrito Leste da Secretaria de Saúde do Município de Campinas/SP. O projeto de doutorado em questão, trata da análise da implementação desde serviço na visão dos usuários. A própria pesquisadora entrará em contato com os potenciais voluntários a serem escolhidos aleatoriamente dentre aqueles que já concluíram suas próteses dentais, aqueles que estão em processo de confecção de próteses e aqueles que ainda aguardam uma vaga na "lista de espera" das Unidades Básicas de Saúde. [...] O tamanho da amostra não é relevante pois trata-se de uma pesquisa que privilegia a análise qualitativa em que a representatividade amostral em relação ao universo pesquisado não é considerada. O principal é aprofundamento da informação e este se dá menos na quantidade de pessoas entrevistadas e mais

Endereço: Rua Tessália Vieira de Camargo, 126
Bairro: Barão Geraldo   **CEP:** 13.083-887
UF: SP   **Município:** CAMPINAS
Telefone: (19)3521-8936   **Fax:** (19)3521-7187   **E-mail:** cep@fcm.unicamp.br

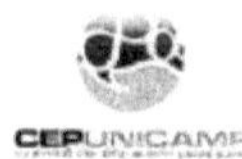

COMITÊ DE ÉTICA EM PESQUISA DA UNICAMP - CAMPUS CAMPINAS

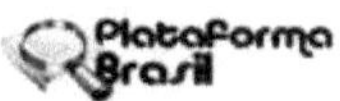

nas estratégias de obter tais informações. No decorrer de todas pesquisa não serão revelados nomes das pessoas envolvidas, nem endereços/contatos que possam vir a identifica-las. Espera-se identificar as dimensões subjetivas dos pacientes mutilados dentais, compreendendo o processo de trabalho, dentro do contexto vigente, analisando as potencialidades e as dificuldades na ótica dos sujeitos/pacientes, apontando possibilidades instituintes de qualificação do serviço."

Considerações sobre os Termos de apresentação obrigatória:

Foram apresentados:

1.Folha de rosto devidamente assinada e datada.

2.Projeto de pesquisa

3.Formulário de informações básicas do projeto na Plataforma Brasil

4.TCLE

5.Carta de autorização

6.Roteiro de entrevista

7.Comprovante de vínculo

8.Cronograma

9.Carta resposta

Conclusões ou Pendências e Lista de Inadequações:

Lista de pendências e inadequações não atendidas emitidas no parecer CEP Nº1.626.764:

4) Adequar o TCLE conforme disposto nos itens sobre Avaliação de riscos e benefícios e sobre os Termos de apresentação obrigatória acima. Resposta: Foi anexado um novo TCLE Análise: A pesquisadora precisa complementar as informações sobre os áudios gravados no item procedimentos: Sobre o destino dos áudios gravados durante as sessões de entrevistas: Serão armazenados? Se sim, por quanto tempo? Como serão descartados? Pretende-se usar em projetos futuros ou será utilizado exclusivamente para este projeto? Pendência parcialmente atendida.

Resposta: O TCLE não contempla as informações solicitadas. A versão atual (modeloTCLErespostapendencia020716.pdf 02/07/2016 11:43:26) contempla a seguinte informação: " Participando do estudo você será convidado para agendar uma entrevista que será gravada em áudio e terá duração de 30 a 40 minutos. Nesta entrevista serão abordados temas relativos à sua saúde bucal. Será combinado um local adequando de sua escolha para realizar a entrevista".

Análise: Pendência não atendida

Resposta:As entrevistas não serão armazenadas após a conclusão da pesquisa e não serão

Endereço: Rua Tessália Vieira de Camargo, 126
Bairro: Barão Geraldo   **CEP:** 13.083-887
UF: SP   **Município:** CAMPINAS
Telefone: (19)3521-8936   **Fax:** (19)3521-7187   **E-mail:** cep@fcm.unicamp.br

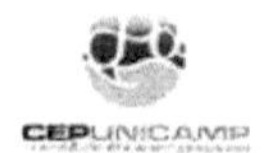

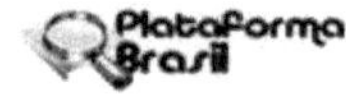

Continuação do Parecer: 1.668.950

utilizadas em novas pesquisas. Foi inserido um novo Termo de Consentimento Livre e Esclarecido informando que ao final da pesquisa as entrevistas serão destruídas.
Análise:Pendência Atendida.

7) Ainda não ficou claro se haverá participação de menores de idade na pesquisa. Ao discorrer sobre os mutilados dentais, há um grande foco em crianças. Fica assim a dúvida se os entrevistados serão ou não crianças/adolescentes. Em caso positivo, o TCLE deve ser direcionado aos pais e deverá ser anexado o termo de assentimento para os menores de idade. Em pesquisas cujos convidados sejam adolescentes, é necessário à anuência do participante da pesquisa através do termo de assentimento livre esclarecido, sem prejuízo do consentimento de seus responsáveis legais. Tais participantes devem ser esclarecidos sobre a natureza da pesquisa, seus objetivos, métodos, benefícios previstos, potenciais riscos e o incômodo que esta possa lhes acarretar, na medida de sua compreensão e respeitados em suas singularidades.
Resposta: Não localizamos a resposta a esta pendência.
Análise: Pendência não atendida
Resposta:Segundo informações contempladas na carta resposta anexada: "Após discussão com a orientadora, ficou decidido que serão incluídos na pesquisa somente participantes acima de 18 anos. Com isso, não será necessário aplicar o termo de assentimento. Essa informação foi incluída no projeto detalhado".
Análise:Pendência Atendida.

Considerações Finais a critério do CEP:
- O sujeito de pesquisa deve receber uma via do Termo de Consentimento Livre e Esclarecido, na íntegra, por ele assinado (quando aplicável).

- O sujeito da pesquisa tem a liberdade de recusar-se a participar ou de retirar seu consentimento em qualquer fase da pesquisa, sem penalização alguma e sem prejuízo ao seu cuidado (quando aplicável).

- O pesquisador deve desenvolver a pesquisa conforme delineada no protocolo aprovado. Se o pesquisador considerar a descontinuação do estudo, esta deve ser justificada e somente ser realizada após análise das razões da descontinuidade pelo CEP que o aprovou. O pesquisador deve aguardar o parecer do CEP quanto à descontinuação, exceto quando perceber risco ou dano não

Endereço: Rua Tessália Vieira de Camargo, 126
Bairro: Barão Geraldo   **CEP:** 13.083-887
UF: SP   **Município:** CAMPINAS
Telefone: (19)3521-8936   **Fax:** (19)3521-7187   **E-mail:** cep@fcm.unicamp.br

Continuação do Parecer: 1.668.950

previsto ao sujeito participante ou quando constatar a superioridade de uma estratégia diagnóstica ou terapêutica oferecida a um dos grupos da pesquisa, isto é, somente em caso de necessidade de ação imediata com intuito de proteger os participantes.

- O CEP deve ser informado de todos os efeitos adversos ou fatos relevantes que alterem o curso normal do estudo. É papel do pesquisador assegurar medidas imediatas adequadas frente a evento adverso grave ocorrido (mesmo que tenha sido em outro centro) e enviar notificação ao CEP e à Agência Nacional de Vigilância Sanitária – ANVISA – junto com seu posicionamento.

- Eventuais modificações ou emendas ao protocolo devem ser apresentadas ao CEP de forma clara e sucinta, identificando a parte do protocolo a ser modificada e suas justificativas e aguardando a aprovação do CEP para continuidade da pesquisa. Em caso de projetos do Grupo I ou II apresentados anteriormente à ANVISA, o pesquisador ou patrocinador deve enviá-las também à mesma, junto com o parecer aprovatório do CEP, para serem juntadas ao protocolo inicial.

- Relatórios parciais e final devem ser apresentados ao CEP, inicialmente seis meses após a data deste parecer de aprovação e ao término do estudo.

-Lembramos que segundo a Resolução 466/2012 , item XI.2 letra e, "cabe ao pesquisador apresentar dados solicitados pelo CEP ou pela CONEP a qualquer momento".

Este parecer foi elaborado baseado nos documentos abaixo relacionados:

Tipo Documento	Arquivo	Postagem	Autor	Situação
Informações Básicas do Projeto	PB_INFORMAÇÕES_BÁSICAS_DO_P ROJETO_653260.pdf	04/08/2016 14:31:25		Aceito
Projeto Detalhado / Brochura Investigador	doutorado_com_consertos_p_CEP_040 82016.pdf	04/08/2016 14:30:47	Ana Cláudia Moutella Pimenta Giudice	Aceito
TCLE / Termos de Assentimento / Justificativa de Ausência	modelo_TCLE_resposta_pendencia_04_ 08_16.pdf	04/08/2016 14:25:24	Ana Cláudia Moutella Pimenta Giudice	Aceito
Outros	Carta_Resposta_ao_Comite_de_Ética_	04/08/2016	Ana Cláudia	Aceito

Endereço: Rua Tessália Vieira de Camargo, 126
Bairro: Barão Geraldo   **CEP:** 13.083-887
UF: SP   **Município:** CAMPINAS
Telefone: (19)3521-8936   **Fax:** (19)3521-7187   **E-mail:** cep@fcm.unicamp.br

Outros	em_Pesquisa_2.pdf	14:24:46	Moutella Pimenta Giudice	Aceito
Declaração de Instituição e Infraestrutura	Declaracaodaintituicao.pdf	02/07/2016 11:49:26	Ana Cláudia Moutella Pimenta Giudice	Aceito
Outros	Roteiro_Entrevista.pdf	02/05/2016 13:14:32	Ana Cláudia Moutella Pimenta Giudice	Aceito
Folha de Rosto	folhaderosto.pdf	14/02/2016 11:56:32	Ana Cláudia Moutella Pimenta Giudice	Aceito
Outros	carteirinha.pdf	10/02/2016 08:53:21	Ana Cláudia Moutella Pimenta Giudice	Aceito
Cronograma	Cronograma.pdf	18/01/2016 13:54:50	Ana Cláudia Moutella Pimenta Giudice	Aceito

Situação do Parecer:
Aprovado

Necessita Apreciação da CONEP:
Não

CAMPINAS, 09 de Agosto de 2016

Assinado por:
Renata Maria dos Santos Celeghini
(Coordenador)

Interview Script

A)SEMI STRUCTURED INTERVIEW

The aim of this interview is to retrieve the interviewee's life story prior to his tooth loss. To this end, we will look at his experiences with oral health care during three phases of his life: childhood, adolescence and adulthood.

Each phase will be defined chronologically by the interviewee. We will be looking for narratives related to oral health care. How they took care of it, who they took care of, if they remember any significant events. We will ask the interviewees about their perceptions of going to a health service.

B)OPEN Interview

We will leave the interviewee as free as possible to narrate their experiences. We will only intervene when we need any clarification regarding speech, expression, gestures...

"Since you lost your teeth, what has happened in your life?"

Timeline:

First semester 2014:

Completion of compulsory courses

Diary construction

Reading/studying themes/articles associated with the topic

Second half of 2014:

Completion of compulsory courses

Continuing to build the diary

Reading/studying themes/articles associated with the topic

First semester 2015:

Completion of compulsory courses

Continuing to build the diary

Reading/studying themes/articles associated with the topic

Start of thesis writing

Second half of 2015:

Completion of compulsory courses

Continuing to build the diary

Reading/studying themes/articles associated with the topic

Suitability of the thesis writing for submission to the Ethics Committee

First semester 2016:

Completion of compulsory courses

Continuing to build the diary

Reading/studying themes/articles associated with the topic

Submission to the Ethics Committee

Fieldwork - Interviews with users

Second half of 2016:

Continuing to build the diary and starting the analysis

Reading/studying themes/articles associated with the topic

Transcription of interviews

Thesis qualification

First semester 2017:

Continuation of diary construction and analysis

Post-qualification corrections/adjustments

Construction of discussions and analysis

Second half of 2017:

Continuation of diary construction and analysis

Continuation of post-qualification corrections/adjustments

Continuation of the discussion and analysis Defense of the thesis

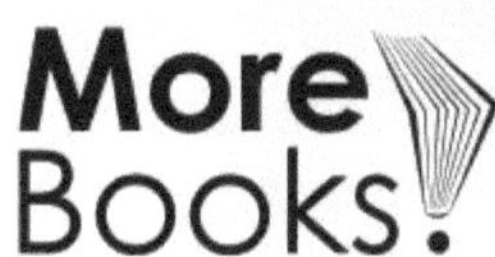

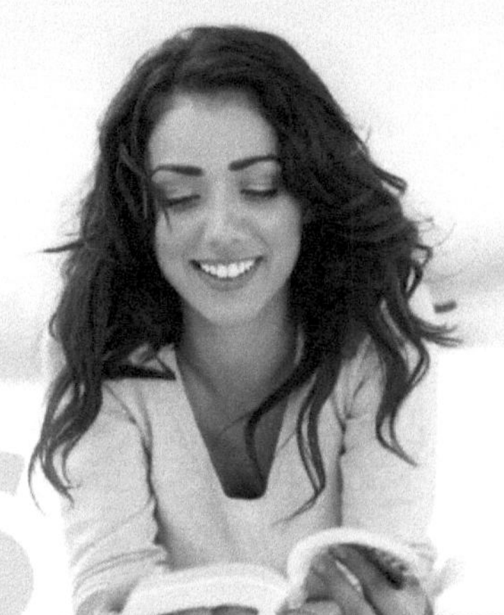

yes
I want morebooks!

Buy your books fast and straightforward online - at one of world's fastest growing online book stores! Environmentally sound due to Print-on-Demand technologies.

Buy your books online at
www.morebooks.shop

Kaufen Sie Ihre Bücher schnell und unkompliziert online – auf einer der am schnellsten wachsenden Buchhandelsplattformen weltweit! Dank Print-On-Demand umwelt- und ressourcenschonend produzi ert.

Bücher schneller online kaufen
www.morebooks.shop

info@omniscriptum.com
www.omniscriptum.com

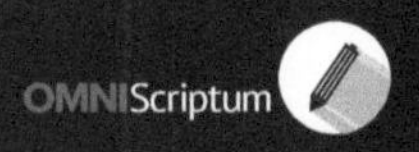

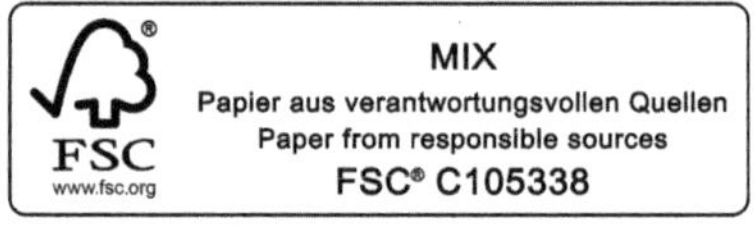

Printed by Books on Demand GmbH, Norderstedt / Germany